KITCHEN MEDICINE

KITCHEN MEDICINE

How I Fed My Daughter
out of Failure to Thrive

DEBI LEWIS

ROWMAN & LITTLEFIELD
Lanham • Boulder • New York • London

Published by Rowman & Littlefield
An imprint of The Rowman & Littlefield Publishing Group, Inc.
4501 Forbes Boulevard, Suite 200, Lanham, Maryland 20706
www.rowman.com

86-90 Paul Street, London EC2A 4NE, United Kingdom

British Library Cataloguing in Publication Information Available

Library of Congress Cataloging-in-Publication Data

Names: Lewis, Debi, 1974- author.
Title: Kitchen medicine : how I fed my daughter out of failure to thrive /
    Debi Lewis.
Description: Lanham : Rowman & Littlefield, [2022] | Includes index.
Identifiers: LCCN 2021046369 (print) | LCCN 2021046370 (ebook) | ISBN
    9781538156650 (cloth) | ISBN 9781538156667 (epub)
Subjects: LCSH: Medicine, Popular. | Traditional medicine. | Kitchens.
Classification: LCC RC82 .L47 2022 (print) | LCC RC82 (ebook) | DDC
    615.8/8—dc23/eng/20211028
LC record available at https://lccn.loc.gov/2021046369
LC ebook record available at https://lccn.loc.gov/2021046370

♾️™ The paper used in this publication meets the minimum requirements of
American National Standard for Information Sciences—Permanence of Paper
for Printed Library Materials, ANSI/NISO Z39.48-1992.

Dedicated to Ronni Lewis. Always.

CONTENTS

INTRODUCTION

I began writing this book while staring out the window of a coffee shop. It was an autumn day and, though I didn't know it yet, the most painful part of my story was over. Sammi had been without her medication for four days. She ate two blueberry muffins that morning, warm out of the oven, eagerly and between snatches of joyful chatter. As we made our way down the alley alongside our house toward her early morning chorus practice, she was an unremarkably normal child, holding the last bites of muffin in her hand and telling me nine-year-old truths as the autumn leaves fell around her.

Before she was born, I couldn't have guessed at the ingredient list for a muffin, let alone *this* muffin, a muffin I'd come to make after years of adapting it in half a dozen other ways: tiny, enormous, without gluten and dairy, without fat, with egg substitutes, and on and on. This one, this favorite muffin being popped bite by bite into the mouth of this little girl I'd struggled to feed at all, was—for me, if not for her—a talisman of our journey together.

So, too, was the coffee shop window where I sat to write. For almost nine years, I'd been coming to this coffee shop and ordering variations of the same espresso drink and eating the same warm cranberry and pecan scone from my window seat. There was crucial peace for me in the ritual of setting out my laptop and mouse, plugging in my headphones, and then pivoting to take my favorite breakfast from Dex, the bearded, smiling barista who had been handing me that scone for all the years of my learning to feed my child. To loosen my ears from my shoulders after a morning of wrangling calories into my younger daughter, I needed all of it: the window seat, the sweet espresso drink, Dex's smile, and the warm scone, each bite in my mouth full of the chew of

1

dried cranberries and the gentle crunch of nuts. Some days, the man who made the scones delivered them later than usual, and I sipped my drink slowly as I waited for him to arrive, his plastic tub of baked goods and fresh bananas perched on the top of his head as he walked past my window. I paid ahead for that scone. It was a sacrament for my workday.

Food has always meant more than just fuel to me, but that truth became clearer when Sammi was born in 2005. For the first nine years of her life, the question of how to keep her nourished—how to feed my way out of that reproachful "failure to thrive" label that topped her medical chart—occupied an enormous part of my churning mind. Her constant medical problems and seeming inability to eat centered on issues with swallowing, and every solution proposed to me had something to do with the space between my stove and my refrigerator. There was medicine, of course, and there were surgeries and doctor's appointments and therapies and consultations, but more than anything else, there was food—rules and structure and complicated diets, restrictions and extra calories, so many changes I can mark those years by food-related phases. I don't know what it was during all those years that kept me from turning on food, from hating it and resenting it, but instead of never wanting to look at the stove again, I kept returning, curious and seeking joy and wonder.

And even when I thought I couldn't mix another starch with another protein, my escape was usually also into food, the greatest comforts being the foods someone else made for me or that I bought, alone, just for me, the scones in the coffee shop window and the tub of cherries at the farmers market, the glass casserole dish of stewed lentils my friend Christine brought me when I had the flu. Even the drive-through hot cocoa, sipped in the front seat as Sammi slept in the back, fed more than my thirst; it fed my need for care and indulgence, my comfort and sweetness when I felt so alone.

When it was all over, when we were without restriction and could eat anywhere and anything we wanted, I still came back to my kitchen. There was something about the process, from raw ingredients and googled recipes to finished product that did more than just feed Sammi and me. It satisfied me in a way that nothing else could, the expertise I'd nurtured giving birth to joy. A blueberry muffin recipe, honed and curated, came from the contributions of farmers and chefs and cookbook authors and my friends; the patience to try and try again, to believe it would be delicious someday, came from a wellspring that seemed, somehow, to have no end. On this journey to becoming nourished, what I discovered about cooking and feeding the people I love has changed everything.

1

HOT CHOCOLATE,
FROZEN IN PLACE

When my second daughter, Sammi, was born, I could barely cook. Seven years before, when my husband David and I had first moved in together after our wedding, I'd called my mother on the phone, horrified by the prospect of making dinner every night.

"How do you do this?" I'd groaned, staring at the one cookbook someone had given me as a wedding gift.

"Well, what did you eat before you got married?" she asked me.

I was embarrassed to tell her about my single-woman eating habits: some nights, I stopped at the White Hen Pantry and bought a pound-sized tub of tapioca pudding, which I ate in noisy slurps in front of the TV. If I felt guilty about not eating vegetables for several days, I'd make couscous and then dump in a can of mixed vegetables along with some butter and a big handful of powdered parmesan cheese. Most nights, though, I just melted cheddar cheese on some tortilla chips and called it a night.

Of course, David actually didn't care if I cooked dinner every night, but I felt like this was the next logical step on my path to becoming an adult. My mother had always made dinner and so had his; I absorbed the matriarchal duty on my own. Someday, I reasoned, there would be children to feed, and I'd witnessed David trying to bake a potato in the oven during the course of many hours with minimal success. Partially due to gender norms and partially due to feeling—at least marginally—the most qualified of the two of us, I subscribed to *Vegetarian Times* magazine and started clipping recipes into a small black plastic binder. It was slow going, but eventually I could make a few simple meals whenever we didn't lazily wander down to the Le Sabre Diner for greasy egg-and-cheese sandwiches on English muffins for $2.50 a piece.

When our first daughter, Ronni, was born, though, I got more serious. My mom taught me to make my own baby food with an immersion blender, and when I was whizzing up broccoli or pears or green beans for her, I saved some of the non-whizzed vegetables for us, finding new ways to use them. Ronni was a voracious eater, excited about everything, earning herself the nickname "owl baby" because of the way she craned her head nearly 180 degrees while sitting in the little high chair that clipped to our kitchen table, excited to catch a glimpse of dinner as soon as she possibly could.

In general, food delighted her. Her day-care provider told us she could polish off a can of beans almost by herself at ten months. Things began appearing on my grocery list that we'd never bought before: beans, of course, but also the ingredients for thick, creamy egg salad; fresh corn on the cob; tubs of strawberries; graham crackers. By then, the raging lactose intolerance I'd developed after my first year of marriage (goodbye, tubs of tapioca pudding and egg-and-cheese sandwiches) finally was met with the arrival of passable—if not amazing—dairy-free cheese substitutes, which I sprinkled liberally on almost everything.

By the time Ronni was a year and a half old, I'd started serving her all the simple meals I'd learned to make: pasta with sautéed mushrooms, steamed broccoli, and sun-dried tomatoes; stir-fried vegetables and seitan (a faux meat I'd tried at a Chinese restaurant and hunted down at a fancy health food store); frozen macaroni and cheese with peas mixed in; tortillas with refried beans and sautéed peppers. She loved to eat. David's mother, Susan, gathered the rest of the family around to watch when we approached her with a spoon; Ronni so loved food that she opened her mouth comically wide, her little feet kicking happily under her seat.

She ate absolutely everything we offered her. One day at a restaurant, I'd pulled the onions off my sandwich and laid them on the side of my plate. When my back was turned, she reached over, grabbed a glistening strip of onion, and stuffed it in her mouth. We howled with laughter as we watched her react to it, and then laughed even harder when she reached for another. She was the same way with everything, clutching rice cakes to her chest, gobbling up big chunks of fresh pears, gleefully learning to spoon yogurt into her mouth. She grew strong and healthy, red cheeked and curious and tremendously fun to feed.

So, two years later, when her little sister Sammi was born, I hadn't given any thought to our eventual introduction of solid foods. I was worried about the sleep deprivation of her first months and the way she might affect Ronni's life. I was worried about doubling the cost of day care. I was worried about how I could possibly love her as much as I loved Ronni. But when Sammi arrived by emergency C-section after a traumatic day of medical interventions, how I would feed her was the last thing on my mind.

To our surprise, she was less than five pounds despite being a week past her due date. When a nurse finally handed her to me in the recovery room after surgery, I was worried that she might not be able to breastfeed. After all, Ronni and I had struggled with breastfeeding for the first month, and she'd been nearly a pound bigger. When I put Sammi to my breast, though, the strength of her suckle made me gasp. From such a tiny mouth, I expected a feeble latch and a lot of frustration. Instead, she was fierce and attached. Shaped like a little doll, she was a perfect baby in miniature. She nursed contentedly until, seemingly in mid-swallow, she was pulled from my arms by a nurse who told me, almost as an aside as my skin cooled where Sammi had been laying, that Sammi had a blood sugar regulation issue that required time in the ICU. I cried as they took her away.

Despite Sammi's immediate ease with nursing, there were hurdles to feeding in that first week. Her nurses argued that her blood sugar issue made her too tired to suckle. They said feeding her via her nasogastric tube (known colloquially as an NG tube) would be easier for her. When I finally convinced them to let me try breastfeeding her—after begging the nurses on the maternity ward to wheel me to the ICU two floors away—the process was ghastly.

First, a nurse would weigh her. Next, I would breastfeed her, and the nurse would weigh her again. Once these numbers were recorded, the nurse would calmly remove the end of Sammi's NG tube from where it was taped to the side of her face, insert a suction plunger into the end, suck all the milk through the tube out of Sammi's stomach, measure it, and then force it back through the NG tube again. There was a radical contrast between peaceful moments of nursing—the rush of love I felt, Sammi's fluttering eyelids and the way she melted into my arms—and the invasive, almost violent suctioning of her stomach. I couldn't wait for her blood sugar to stabilize so I could get her home, away from this eat-suction-refeed cycle.

Despite the intense focus on Sammi's nutrient intake, I don't remember much at all about what I ate during those first few weeks, and no one else seemed to be paying attention to me, either. I was instructed to guzzle water to help my milk come in, which I did through a straw protruding from the ridiculous beer stein–shaped plastic mug the hospital sent home with me. In an effort to sustain my daughter, I drank so much water that I gagged as the nurse wagged her finger at me, scolding me for finishing only two of the thirty-ounce cups that day. It seemed that if it benefited Sammi, it was worth pressing it on me. The fact that I'd been accidentally served a tuna sandwich despite my deadly seafood allergy was met with little more than a shrug as the nurse walked out of the room.

Even after we brought Sammi home, a growing sense of unease made the days and then the weeks blend together, leaving my own needs just barely met. Somehow, I must have gotten Ronni fed once David went back to work, but photographs of me from that time reveal that I lost the pregnancy weight so quickly that my hair fell out. Perhaps it was the worry combined with the utter lack of sleep. Sammi was nothing like Ronni as an infant. When Sammi slept—which was rare and in thirty-minute bursts—she made a ghastly sound, a rasping, wet gurgle that grew louder each week. A visit to a pediatric otolaryngologist revealed floppy tissue in her throat and gastrointestinal reflux. When I tried to go back to work after three months, that sound turned, one terrifying night, into a horrible respiratory infection that saw me racing the four miles to the hospital, reaching back to jiggle the car seat until she made a sound, afraid the whole way that she had stopped breathing. She was prescribed steroids and given breathing treatments and sent home the next morning, leaving David and me shocked and exhausted. Ronni, at age three, never had needed even an antibiotic.

A month later, it happened again, and this time, it was more than a night in the hospital. Sammi was admitted for five days. I was not allowed to nurse her; her breathing was so labored, she'd have aspirated the milk, leading to a lung infection. They inserted an IV to keep her hydrated, and each time David came to relieve me, I would escape to the other side of the room with my breast pump, anxious to keep my supply up. In the pouch of my breast pump bag was a supply of apples and granola bars, all I had to sustain me during the long hours of the day when David was gone.

Not being able to nurse Sammi left me feeling useless. In the four months since her birth, she'd gained almost seven pounds, all on my milk. I was proud of this and, what's more, my growing feelings of guilt over not feeling as connected to her as I was to Ronni had been quieted daily by that intimacy. Her eagerness to nurse was my reassurance that she needed me. I'd relished the rush of oxytocin—the "love hormone"—that accompanied my milk letdown. Holding Sammi in my arms, feeling her body relax as she nursed, was the closest I'd come to communing with her. I didn't know what was wrong with her breathing. I didn't know why she barely slept. I didn't know how to fix the ache I saw in her eyes, a plea for rescue I couldn't fully grasp, but I could nurse her, and that was sometimes enough.

Now, I felt utterly defeated, holding her in my arms in the hospital room, helplessly refusing her the one thing she wanted most. As I rocked, bounced, held, and worried about her, I felt myself and my own needs floating away. I had to pee, to eat, and to sleep, but none of those things happened on my schedule anymore. I'd brought my GRE study book with me, thinking I'd practice logic problems for my upcoming exam while she slept, but there were few opportunities for that. In my all-encompassing worry, there wasn't even time for my frustration.

A few hours after David left on our fourth night in the hospital, Sammi began to cry with a new intensity. Without nursing in my tool kit, I tried singing, rocking, dancing, petting, whispering in her ear, and walking the room. Nothing worked. Nurses and families passing by her room looked curiously at us: a sweating, bedraggled mother and her screaming, frantic baby.

After an hour, I was sure something new was wrong. To the nurse who came to monitor her vital signs, I said, "I wonder if something is hurting her."

The nurse brusquely looked in her ears again, checked her diaper, and told me not to worry. She shut the door behind her as I resumed my shuffle around the room, Sammi screaming into my shoulder.

My ears had begun to hurt from the volume of her cries, so I carefully maneuvered her into the sling again, trailing wires and cords. I wore a path between the bed and the crib, the chair and the wall. Several times, I collapsed into a wide-legged seated position, my eleven-pound four-month-old tight against my chest, and tried to determine whether her cries were louder or unchanged.

Desperately alone, I panicked, silently. By ten o'clock at night, nearly two hours into this unbroken misery, the nurse told me again that there was nothing wrong with Sammi. I burst into tears.

Her face softened slightly, and she put her hand authoritatively on my shoulder. "Come on, Mom," she said firmly. "You have another child. You know babies cry sometimes, and we don't always know why."

"But this isn't like her," I pleaded. "This is a different cry. I don't know how to help her."

"I have an idea," the nurse said, peering up at the television. "Have you ever tried one of those Baby Einstein videos?"

Momentarily, I was too angry to be distraught. The insanity of this suggestion—that a four-month-old baby would shriek like this due to boredom—left me speechless. Still, I let her try. In a series of surreal moments, I pointed at the screen and narrated for Sammi. *It's a bear! Look at the bear!*

She cried on, never opening her eyes. Soaked against my chest in the sling, she seemed utterly unaware of anything outside the tiny universe of whatever she was feeling. We paced the room to the tune of the xylophone music on the screen for another ten minutes, after which I turned it off and finally contributed a soundtrack of my own sobs, moaning, *I'm sorry I can't help you. I'm sorry you're so sad. I'm so sorry. I'm so sorry.*

The nurse closed the door to the hallway, which she'd accidentally left open, complaining that we were keeping the other patients from sleeping.

At midnight, a new nurse came on shift. She came into our room where I was pacing with Sammi, who was still wrapped in a sling on my chest, crying and clutching my shirt in her free hand. I had one hand on the IV pole and another patting her bottom. My lips were pressed against the top of her ear, no longer shushing or singing, only murmuring nonsense, utterly shattered. The new nurse took one look at us, closed the door gently behind her, sat in the chair by the side of the bed, and said, "I hear you've been having a rough night."

"Yes," I said, out of tears and over the sound of Sammi's continued cries, which by now were getting softer as she lost her voice. "I don't know what to do. She's never been like this before, not ever."

"Well," the nurse said, never taking her eyes off us, "you know, she's been on IV fluids for days now, so she's hydrated and getting some nutrition through that, but her tummy still might feel empty. We might be able to try giving her a bottle. Do you have any expressed breastmilk?"

"Yes!" I said. "Yes, it's in the fridge down the hall. It's labeled with her name."

"Why don't you let me hold her while you get some? I can give her a bottle; maybe she'd be more likely to take it from me."

I eased Sammi out of the sling, careful to hold the IV tubing and monitor leads away, and placed her, still howling, into the arms of the nurse. Before I could reach the door of the room, the nurse said from behind me, "Wait. When was her IV last checked?"

"I don't know," I said, turning to face her. "Don't they do that when they check her vitals?"

The nurse was removing the splint around Sammi's IV as I answered, and she interrupted. "Go to the nursing station right now and bring me two more nurses. Tell them we have an infiltration."

"What is that?" I asked.

"They'll know. Just go right away," she answered, laying Sammi on the bed. With the empty sling still dangling from my neck, I did as she asked, and when the nurses I found heard why they were needed, they leaped up and ran to our room.

What was happening was indeed alarming. Sammi's IV needle had infiltrated the tissue of her arm.

Intravenous infiltration occurs when the needle bringing fluids into a patient's vein comes out of the vein and into the surrounding tissue. Instead of the fluid from the IV bag entering the patient's bloodstream, it enters the area under the skin, spreading further and further as long as fluid continues to flow through the needle. It can happen the moment an IV is inserted, or it can happen afterward due to a change in position or extra-tight tape or just bad luck.

Sammi's IV probably had infiltrated sometime around 8:30 p.m. The nursing shift change happened at midnight, so Sammi likely had IV fluid—in her case, a combination of saline and dextrose—entering the tissues of her arm the whole time. When the nurse removed the splint around her IV, Sammi's hand and arm were swollen with fluid from the tips of her fingers almost all the way to her armpit. Her hand was so swollen that her fingers were stuck together. The skin of her wrist had begun to split. When the new nurse removed the IV and applied a warm compress, Sammi stopped crying almost instantly, looked up at me, and smiled. Moments later, she fell asleep in my arms. I watched in horror as yellow droplets of IV fluid began bubbling up through the skin of her arm.

I had no idea, then, that what had happened was the result of negligence. I put the bottle of pumped breastmilk on the bedside table, forgetting I'd even brought it from the refrigerator until the next morning when I found it curdled there. I couldn't focus. I was soaked in sweat—as was Sammi—and so wrecked from more than three hours of begging for someone to take me seriously that the only thing I could do was climb into the hospital bed, tuck Sammi into the crook of my arm, and fall into a heavy sleep.

In the morning, the nurses told me they had stopped by every hour all night long to shine a flashlight in Sammi's eyes, take her temperature, and replace the warm packs on her arm. We had both slept through it all.

No new IV was inserted during the remainder of that hospital stay. Instead, slow-flow nipples were fitted to the bottles of breastmilk I'd pumped, and she drank my milk again. Though she crooked her neck hard against my chest, trying to nurse instead of bottle-feed, eventually her hunger got the best of her, and she managed the bottles, barely. It was not lost on me that my inability to breastfeed her as I'd wanted was what led the nurse to hold her and discover the problem.

Can no one effectively feed this baby? I thought.

A few weeks later, Sammi turned five months old, and I said goodbye to all my coworkers as I resigned myself to staying home full time. After we'd called the pediatric otolaryngologist to describe this recent hospital stay, he strongly suggested that we keep Sammi away from other people until she outgrew that floppy bit of tissue in her throat, which would make every virus result in another admission to the hospital.

"She's going to get sick like this every time, I'm afraid," he'd told me over the phone when I called. "You're better off keeping her home until she outgrows it. I'd hate to see her end up with multiple rounds of pneumonia, or worse."

So I quit my job, my only tether to the outside world. For the rest of that winter, Sammi continued to sleep in her tiny power naps only, day and night. I zombied my way through the days at home, *Mary Poppins* on repeat for Ronni after her afternoon nap as Sammi marathon-nursed through the hours between three and five, attached to my nipple on the couch as I dozed in and out of sleep, alert for anything Ronni might need. Some days, as I sat being drained dry by this tiny baby, I realized dreamily that I could not remember when or what I'd last eaten. I could remember the Cream of Wheat I'd made Ronni for breakfast and the caffeine-free soda I'd drank first thing that morning. Did I have a bagel maybe? Did I grab a handful of dry cereal? *I need to eat something as soon as she's done,* I'd tell myself, but then Sammi would fall asleep in my lap, and I wouldn't want to put her down again.

For months, my only real culinary joy was the soy-milk hot chocolate I'd order from the only drive-through Starbucks for miles around, twenty minutes from the preschool Ronni attended a few days a week. It was almost the only time I left the house. After Sammi and I dropped Ronni off, I'd drive until Sammi was asleep, circling the block around Starbucks. I'd had a peppermint version of this drink at least five days a week during my pregnancy with Sammi, the mint cutting through my mild nausea every morning and the milk adding enough protein that I didn't feel guilty about the cookie I usually ate along with it. Sometimes I held the cup in both hands on my walk from Starbucks into the office, holding it up to my face just to breathe in the scent of peppermint, my queasiness dissipating with every step.

(Three years later, wild spearmint grew between the cracks in the pavement of our backyard. Sammi, two years old, loved it so much that she would pull leaves off to chew whenever she passed it. In the coming years, she would love everything mint: ice cream, cookies, even lemonade with mint leaves. Marveling as my four-year-old sipped unsweetened mint tea at the kitchen counter, I wondered if my obsession during pregnancy had planted this flavor preference in her.)

But during her first winter, I drank hot chocolate without the mint, going for full, sweet richness. I'd drive back to the preschool and park while Sammi slept. I brought a book, and as I sipped, I could pretend

I wasn't here: trapped in an endless cycle of nursing and not sleeping; with no job, a rejected application to graduate school, and nothing on the horizon but more of this hazy drudgery.

In fact, soy-milk hot chocolate had been a revelation for me when it launched at Starbucks in 2004, barely more than a year before Sammi was born. The first one I'd tried had hooked me forever—and not just because it was delicious. It hooked me because it meant that someone at some corporate board somewhere had thought about people like me, people watching the Frappuccinoed world go by without us. In a world with much bigger problems, it's a small thing to be able to share a drink at a café with a friend without being compelled to choose a last-resort option—an iced tea to their frothy latte or an iced coffee to their caramel macchiato—but it wore on me. Being left out was something I got used to—a plate of french fries in front of me as my friends gobbled down gooey ice cream sundaes—but it never stopped bothering me. I wanted that frothy, sugary coffee drink. I just wanted it not to make me sick.

When Starbucks started selling drinks made with soy milk, so did other coffee shops. By the time Sammi was older, going in and out of the children's hospital regularly, even the dinky coffee window in the lobby offered soy milk. Being able to get that comforting, silky chocolate drink from a drive-through window—especially during a year in which I watched my husband leaving for work and my friends taking their healthy babies to playgroups and my former coworkers moving on without me and nurses in the hospital calling me *mom* and looking right through me—was a sign from the universe that I mattered. That my needs counted. That my comfort was valuable, somewhere, to some executive who said, *yes, let's offer soy milk*.

Sammi was growing on my breastmilk, despite her inability to sleep well and despite the words "failure to thrive" appearing on a growing number of her medical charts. The label, I knew, had begun to apply to me, too. During a winter when not much else was, that hot chocolate was *good*.

2

BLUEBERRIES, QUARTERED
AND STUCK

By the spring of Sammi's first year, David and I had been forced to come to an understanding about sleep. After I'd become so outrageously overtired during her first two months that I'd passed out on our hardwood floor, we'd hired a postpartum doula to give me respite two nights a week. Unfortunately, when I had to quit my job two months later, that seemed an unreasonable expense, so I'd gone back to waking every sixty to ninety minutes around the clock. Once Sammi's pediatrician had insisted on sleep training for her—three hours or more of Sammi's hysterical, unending screaming every night for three months, an endeavor that thoroughly traumatized me—I slept even more poorly, fitful and anxious. David was working, which meant he needed the quality sleep more than I did. In the end, our agreement was this: on Saturdays, I would get up at dawn with the kids and get them out of the house so he could rest; on Sundays, he did the same for me. In this way, we each got another hour or two of sleep once a week.

In early May, the local farmers market opened. Every Saturday at six in the morning, I buckled both girls into their car seats and hoisted our ridiculous double stroller into the trunk of our car. Just a few miles away, one of the most celebrated markets in the Midwest opened at dawn. On the drive there, I'd suggest to the girls that we "find a rainbow," searching for one fruit or vegetable of each color.

Ronni was four that first summer, with giant brown bottle curls trailing down her back and a love for her little sister that felt, sometimes, far more enthusiastic than my own. In fact, Ronni was more enthusiastic than me about almost everything, especially during that heartaching first year of Sammi's life, full of endless days and nights, nothing ahead but more diapers, more *Mary Poppins*, more half-hearted meals of toast with melted soy cheese and salsa. I kept fruit in the house for the girls, but it had been years since I'd shopped at a farmers market, not since the summer in college when I'd lived in a co-op and it was my job to get the week's order of greens, tomatoes, and fresh eggs. All those years later, taking my daughters to the local market began as an excuse to get out of the house, a place where Sammi might be stimulated enough that she wouldn't scream to leave the stroller. If she did, I'd stuff her into a baby sling against my chest and put our purchases in her seat.

It was at the farmers market where I learned about growing seasons for the first time. In early May, at the first market of the year, we were greeted with a palette of mostly green. We were bundled into winter coats, still, that first year, blankets on the girls' laps. Everywhere were seedlings and the hearty early spring flowers: pots of daffodils and crocuses, tiny plastic carriers for the beginnings of tomatoes and peppers and oregano and romaine lettuce, potential and hope spread across four long rows of booths as I sighed and gave the stroller another shove.

"I see green!" Ronni called again and I reached forward to pet her curls. She wriggled and strained to turn and look up at me. "Mommy, can we grow little green plants?"

Growing kids is plenty, I thought to myself. *Where would I ever find time to grow a pot of herbs? And why?*

More than a decade later, I'd stop next to the Henry's Farm booth to buy pungent basil and feathery anise hyssop plants from the annex his sister Teresa had set up. Having cultivated a relationship with several farmers at the market over the years, I knew how to ask about Genovese versus Thai basil, to pinch the soft leaves of the hyssop and smell the licorice on my fingers. I knew the hyssop would come back year after year and that I was the only one at home who liked it. But in 2005, with my two girls in their sage green stroller, howling and pointing, singing and crying, I didn't give the herb seedlings any consideration; I made straight for the Great Harvest Bread Company stand.

Great Harvest is a franchised bakery, the baked goods they sell in their stores and at their stand at the farmers market boasting a rustic, homemade look. On big trays covered by plastic lids were piles of scones, big blueberry muffins, and focaccia breads glistening with oil and tomatoes and feta cheese. I wasn't at this stand for myself. I was there for Ronni, who could be content for hours with a pastry. Clutching her giant muffin at age four or her "apple scrapple" bread at age ten, she was always willing to go to the market with me as long as we could stop here. I watched, silently jealous, as she tucked in.

Before Ronni was born, it had become increasingly clear to me that my lactose intolerance was getting worse. The year after David and I were married—the year of the egg-and-cheese sandwiches at Le Sabre Diner—I had all the usual symptoms, quashed by my Wisconsin dairy country upbringing and ignored until I could not ignore them any longer, racing home from the train at the end of the workday to be sick from the cheesy French fries I'd had at lunch. By our first anniversary, I was what I called an "ovo-vegetarian," eating eggs but not dairy products. During my pregnancies, I'd struggled to meet the guidelines on protein consumption, choking down an overly salty-sweet frozen soy product called "rib-lettes" because they had twelve grams per serving. Restaurants were a challenge; bakeries were a taunting, teasing trial of my will to prioritize my health. I missed the enormous muffins and the heavy scones of my lactose tolerant years.

And now, week after week, I watched as my voracious, mini-epicurean daughter ate all the baked goods I couldn't. During the early spring weeks of the market, the ready-to-eat options were limited: fresh, raw mushrooms from the mushroom farmer; super-pricey bags of dried cranberries from the farm that also sold preserves and jams; or raw radishes. They were hardly what I wanted at six or seven in the morning— or, in the case of the cranberries, what I felt justified in purchasing at all at their exorbitant price. The first few weeks at the market, we saw green and more green, so we had to find the rest of our rainbow in packaging or in the colors of the tents.

By the end of June, though, things always improved rapidly. We started noticing more color each week, starting with strawberries and deep pink raspberries and soon thereafter tomatoes and cherries. I'd buy a small tub of berries right away when we arrived, propping it between the handles of the stroller to nibble as we walked, each bite a surprise— this one tart, this one sweet, this berry firm, this one melting between my tongue and the roof of my mouth. Ronni would hold her hands up in the air, begging for me to place a few berries in her sticky palms. We finished a pint within half an hour.

Everything about berries from the market was different from the berries I'd eaten from the grocery store. I'd always liked strawberries but had come to view them with suspicion. Sometimes they looked beautiful—bright red and glistening—but I'd take a bite and find they were barely flavored at all, a faint taste of strawberry under a watery blandness. I didn't know how to tell when they would be good; there were no clues in the sterile plastic clamshells in the grocery store.

The spring before David and I were married, we'd been invited to a Passover seder at the home of one of his mother's friends. For dessert, they served angel food cake with fresh whole strawberries on top, and I couldn't get enough.

"How did you get strawberries that taste so wonderful?" I asked the hostess.

She'd shrugged at me. "This is when they're good, usually—right around Passover."

It was only the second time in my life I'd been able to associate a food with a season. When I was a little girl, my mother had grown several enormous garden beds of vegetables in our yard in Wisconsin. Most of them, I didn't like—bitter lettuces and sharp onions and hard, crunchy green beans—but every year, the week of July 4, two important things happened out in that garden: my grandfather and his second wife visited and toured it with my mother and the pea pods were ready.

I still don't know the name for the variety of peas my mom grew, but we called them "pea pods." They were probably snow peas—flat and bright green, with a little string we had to pull out unless we wanted it endlessly stuck between our teeth or gagging us when we swallowed. When my mom pronounced the peas ready for eating, my brother and I stood at the edge of the garden bed and leaned forward, holding her metal mixing bowl, and reached for where they'd snaked up the web of string she'd hung. We found the longest, fattest pods and ate them right there, still warm from the sun, until my mother caught us and told us to wash them first, then later we ate them at dinner, just as they were. They didn't taste as good once they'd been stored in the refrigerator; something about the introduction of artificial cold diminished their sweetness.

I remembered that feeling—the sense that there is a flavor in the sun's warmth on fresh food—as I wandered through the market, eating warm strawberries in June with my daughters. One day, buying them from one of the vendors, I asked why they were so good now, when I'd thought strawberries were best in March, near Passover.

"That might be when they're good in Mexico," he answered. "But here in Illinois, strawberries grow in June."

And so now we had green from the still overflowing baskets of herbs and lettuces, kale and chard and spinach and red from the berries and tomatoes and beginnings of chili peppers on tiny manicured bushes for sale. Best of all, we now had blue and purple from the fruit that was about to captivate Sammi: blueberries.

The previous fall, when Sammi was a newborn, my mother-in-law Susan had shown up one Saturday afternoon with a big bag of blueberries from her local farm stand.

"You've got to try these; they're fabulous!" she told us as she put the bag down on our kitchen table. The table was a disaster—newspapers and mail and takeout menus and napkins and baby bottles from David's largely unsuccessful attempts to give me a break from breastfeeding, boxes of cheese-flavored bunny-shaped crackers that Ronni loved, and crumbs and grease we just hadn't found the time to clean up. Thankfully, she overlooked all of that and dug out our colander to wash the berries.

"I'm not such a blueberry fan," I said, holding Sammi against me in the baby sling where, those days, she could be found during all waking hours. I'd never really liked blueberries. They were sour, I thought, and there were those extra-sour seeds in the middle. Even blueberry muffins, I thought, were ruined by the presence of blueberries, sour and mushy and interrupting all that excellent flour and sugar. Ronni had loved them as a baby—she called them "boo-bucks"—but I'd never even tried the ones I bought for her. Why waste them?

"Just try one," Susan pressed.

She was right. These were an entirely different world of blueberry flavor, almost candy-sweet with hints of vanilla and cream. They were firm on the outside and yielded to my teeth with an explosion of juice. I could roll one around in my mouth and taste the skin—the source of the tartness, I realized—and then crush it between my back teeth to extract every other flavor at once.

"Wow," I answered her, my eyes closed a little, hypnotically patting Sammi's bottom as I rocked in place.

So now, ten months later, I bought my first pint of blueberries at my own farmers market. They were just as delicious as the ones Susan had brought us, and now I thought it might be time to let Sammi have some, too.

Sammi had been "eating" solid food for several months by then. Though most pediatricians recommend that babies start to experiment casually with solid food at six months old, ours all but ordered us to get serious about solids when Sammi still had not slept more than two consecutive hours by that age. She had hoped a fuller belly would help Sammi sleep longer. Four months later, Sammi had yet to meet any food with enthusiasm. She'd responded to oatmeal and rice cereal mixed with breastmilk by projectile vomiting in an arc across my kitchen more than once, which the pediatrician told us was a sure sign of grain allergy. For pureed peaches and pears, which had been Ronni's favorites at that age, Sammi would open her mouth in the tiniest O and allow a few molecules at a time to pass her lips. It was only when we resorted to jarred infant food from the grocery store that she showed any enthusiasm for solid food, but even then, she deigned to eat barely half a jar at a time. The only solid food she picked up with her fingers were strange little dehydrated corn kernels that melted into a syrupy ooze once they hit her tongue.

Still, these blueberries were really something special. Maybe the fresh air and the excitement around her would make her hungrier, I thought, and bit one in half, putting the other half on the tray in front of her stroller seat. At first, she poked at it but didn't pick it up, her fine reddish-blond hair blowing across her forehead as she squinted in the sun. I pulled the stroller off to the edge of the market and crouched at her side. This was a long double stroller—one seat in front of the other instead of side by side—and she had the front seat because Ronni's curls had been the subject of her intense grip when we'd tried it the other way.

"Hey Sammi Sunshine," I said to her, one hand brushing her cheek as the other held the pint of blueberries, "these are blueberries. They're really yummy! Want to try one?"

She reached for me, always preferring to be held than to be pushed in the stroller, but I pressed on. I gave a few berries to Ronni, who performed her best babytalk squeak: "Wanna berry, baby Sammi? Baby Sammi wanna yummy boo-berry?"

"You don't have to talk like that, kiddo," I told her. "She can understand your big-kid voice."

"Sammi!" Ronni went on, "These are soooooooo good! Have one!"

I took another blueberry and nibbled half of it away, adding it to the now-mushy half I'd put down before. Sammi finally reached over, pinched one of the halves between her thumb and middle finger, and put it in her mouth.

"*Mmmmm*, right, Sammi?" Ronni cooed.

"*Mmmm mmm!*" Sammi agreed, grinning, her two front teeth already covered with its dark juice. I quickly bit several more berries in half and added them to her tray.

Sammi liked blueberries more than any other food for many, many years. For those first few months, they were almost the only food she would eat on her own with any regularity. I spent time every day carefully cutting blueberries in half (or, if they were too big, in quarters) and putting them in little colorful plastic bowls with lids. At every meal, I'd half-heartedly try to get Sammi to eat something else—refried beans or mashed carrots or some revolting green-beans-and-pear jarred baby food—but she'd refuse. Then I'd bring out the little bowl of blueberry pieces, and she'd coo and reach for them, pushing them into her mouth with one finger.

It bothered me, how little Sammi ate. At nearly a year old, she was still little more than sixteen pounds when the CDC's growth charts suggested the average twelve-month-old baby weighed twenty-one pounds. Even accounting for my size, which is only five feet one, Sammi was still smaller than her older sister at that age by a whole pound. She nursed continually and after a horrible two months of sleep training, she finally slept four or five hours at a time most nights, but she was so very small. There were milestones she simply couldn't meet because of her size—pulling oneself up to a standing position is tough if the coffee table comes up to one's shoulders, for example—and others that seemed like they were tied to never having had textures other than purees in her mouth, like talking. She said "dog" and "duck" and "dada" and "*mmmmmmmmmm*," but that was nothing compared to Ronni, who was babbling to us in multiword phrases by that age, not to mention gumming rice cakes, macaroni and cheese, canned beans, and the occasional peeled apple, which she would hold in both hands and messily press into her face. Sammi had jarred food, dehydrated corn kernels, tiny pieces of watermelon, and halved blueberries. Maybe some of this was totally normal, and I was unreasonably comparing her to her older sister. I didn't know for sure, but something about Sammi's reticence regarding textures and types of food really troubled me. I couldn't put my finger on it.

One rainy summer afternoon, the girls were rolling a ball across our tiled floor when Ronni screamed. "Mommy! There's a bug in Sammi's mouth! *Mommy!*"

I raced over to them and scooped Sammi up in one frenzied movement. Sitting on the edge of the couch, I faced Sammi toward me and held her with one arm while using the fingers of my other hand to force her mouth open. I swept my index finger and thumb around the inside of her mouth as she squirmed and cried.

"I need to see what you ate, Sammi. Stay still," I said calmly through gritted teeth.

When I pulled my fingers out, what I found puzzled me. It was four in the afternoon, hours and a nap since Sammi had eaten lunch. Stuck to my fingers were several blueberry pieces, the skin black against my fingernails.

"Huh," I said aloud.

"Did she eat a bug, Momma?" Ronni asked, still sitting on the tile floor.

"No, no, sweetie," I said, "it's just her blueberries from lunch."

When David came home that night, I told him what I'd found in Sammi's mouth. We were both worried; why was she pouching her food in her cheeks like that? Would that be bad for her teeth? What if she choked on it in her sleep? We agreed to call her pediatrician the next day.

Dr. Lynn was technically Sammi's second pediatrician. Her first had been the same septuagenarian we'd used for Ronni, a man whose demeanor lacked only a clown nose to complete my mental image of him as a performer on autopilot. "Who's two years old today?" he'd sing as he walked into the exam room, drying his freshly washed hands on a paper towel he'd gently toss to the baby to test her reflexes. He'd missed the severity of Sammi's initial floppy tissue diagnosis, rolling his eyes at me when I'd brought her in with rapid breathing and then returned, triumphant, from the specialist with a request for acid reflux medication. He'd never suggested we keep Sammi away from other children, even after she'd been hospitalized for her first cold. On the terrible night when Sammi's most recent respiratory infection was diagnosed—the one that sent us to the hospital where her IV had infiltrated her arm— I'd made an instinctive decision to transfer her care to the pediatrician who'd been on call that day. Dr. Lynn sat with Sammi and me in her office for almost four hours, trying to treat her as an outpatient before finally having her admitted to the hospital down the street. I liked her; she looked me in the eye, didn't talk down to me with platitudes, and always answered my phone calls with a down-to-earth, "Hello, Mrs. Lewis. This is Dr. Lynn. What's going on?"

This time, I apologized before even beginning. "I'm probably being ridiculous," I began. "Ronni was just such an easygoing eater, so maybe my experience is colored by that, but Sammi's eating style is kind of freaking me out."

"How so?"

I explained what had happened the day before. "And, seriously, Dr. Lynn, it was at least three hours—maybe four—since she'd eaten those blueberries. She'd even nursed since then, and they were still all stuffed up inside her cheek. Isn't that weird? Should she be doing that?"

"It's a little weird," she admitted, "but not totally outside the norm. Some kids take longer to take to food. Obviously Sammi has some allergies—that projectile vomiting with the cereal tells us that—but this sounds like it's within the realm of normal. Keep trying, mom. She'll get it."

And so all summer, I pushed our double stroller through the farmers market with Ronni holding her muffin and Sammi and I sharing our tubs of berries. In the heat of July, when stone fruits came into season, Sammi still held out for blueberries. Week after week, I bit them or cut them in half for her, watching to be sure she didn't choke, waiting to be sure she was safe. Week after week, day after day, we tried adding more foods to her diet, throwing them away when she refused. The little green tub of farmers market blueberries was savior and jailer, the only solid food she'd eat with enthusiasm. I was grateful we'd found something but often furious that it was so low in calories.

In some ways, those blueberries became a gateway to our family's appreciation for all kinds of fresh produce. Though the girls and I were vegetarians, we still ate a fairly boring diet composed mostly of simple carbohydrates and a small handful of vegetables: mainly broccoli, peas, and corn. It wasn't that I was unwilling to try new things, but I didn't know where to begin. During the second half of that first summer at the farmers market, a neighbor convinced me to share a weekly box of vegetables from a farm via a CSA (community-supported agriculture) program.

She was a far better cook than I was, and with our first few boxes, I had to ask her what many of the items were. One afternoon, she came to my house to cook with me, teaching me how to strip the leaves off rainbow chard, shred zucchini, and properly crush a clove of garlic with the side of a knife. I was awkward and tentative, but it was hard not to be charmed by the freshness of the foods and their deep, vibrant colors. There was purple lettuce, beets striped like peppermint candy, layers of green inside every leek.

When the carrots arrived, still dusted with dirt from the farm, I was filled, suddenly, with reverence for them. Carrots from the grocery store looked like food, uniformly shaped and sized, in clear plastic bags. These carrots were gnarled and varied, some sporting long skinny tails like hair. Arriving with their frilly green tops attached, I had an unexpected memory of these very frills in my mother's garden and realized that she had been growing carrots. I'd never even realized it.

I tried to imagine how anyone had ever discovered carrots. Centuries ago, someone saw these fronds waving gently above the ground and wondered what lay beneath. That person had to have had enough curiosity to reach down, grab that frond, and pull the long root out of the ground, gently enough not to separate the greens from the carrot itself. Once she saw that root—dirty and strange, flecked with red or purple or orange—she had to have the vision to see it as food. There would have been dirt to brush off and—without the shiny metal peelers we have today—she would have had to break it open to see the bright, wet color inside. After all that, it would have to appeal to her taste. Could she smell it? Did someone lean in, press a nose to the warm dirt surrounding it, and inhale the faint sweetness? Did she lick it, right there, standing in a field or at the edge of a forest? Did she take a small nibble?

Something of that sense of discovery excited me. By the time that summer was over, I felt confident enough to reserve my own weekly box for the next summer. Over the next decade, I would learn how to shred kohlrabi for hash; to peel and cube beets and carrots and potatoes, boil them, and then mix them with mayonnaise and spicy Israeli pickles for my family's favorite summer salad; to sauté all kinds of greens with olive oil and garlic; to panfry halved brussels sprouts to such perfection that Sammi and I would fight over the last one; to chop pounds of heirloom tomatoes and cook them into a thick sauce with bell peppers and garlic and spices to form the base for shakshuka; and to mix fresh basil with raw cashews and garlic and nutritional yeast for a pesto that we froze in quart bags to last all winter.

But it all started with those blueberries. Years later, when Sammi was a little more than thirty pounds upon entering kindergarten, I was tucking her into bed, calling her my little peanut, when she frowned.

"But I don't *like* peanuts," she scowled at me from under her covers.

I explained that it was a term of endearment. "It's a name you call a small person—like a kid—who you think is super cute and who you love so much."

"But *I don't like peanuts*," she insisted.

"Well, what is something small and cute like a peanut that I could call you instead?" I asked her.

She considered it for a moment then smiled. "You could call me your little blueberry!"

I pressed my cheek to the top of her soft, fine hair. "My little blueberry. I love that."

"And I can call you my little peach!" she answered, knowing peaches were my favorite fruit.

There we were, from then on, blueberry and peach, claiming the foods that defined us. From that first tub of blueberries that we shared at the farmers market, we were sweet and tart and sun warmed. Though we were both surrounded by nourishment that we would someday come to cherish, we would be ready for it only in our season.

3

CHICKPEA SOUP,
MY FIRST IMPROVISATION

Sammi turned one in August, and shortly thereafter, a weeklong visit from my best friend Hilary and her congested baby daughter introduced the first serious respiratory infection Sammi had encountered since I'd quit my job nine months before. Within days of them leaving, I returned home from one of my sanity-saving sessions of freelance work at my favorite coffee shop to hear a sound that had been absent from our lives for many months: the rattle and rasp of Sammi with a cold.

When Sammi was sick and struggling to breathe as an infant, we'd done our best to take the advice from the older, condescending male pediatrician who had told us to stop worrying because it was "just a cold." Even when we'd switched to Dr. Lynn, who took us more seriously, we couldn't possibly take Sammi to the doctor every time her breathing was strained; we'd have been there multiple times a week. To keep ourselves from a state of continual panic, we'd come up with several funny nicknames for the breathing that, underneath the jokes, made my whole soul sound an alarm. "Darth Baby" was one moniker, and then there was Ronni's choice: "Baby Snort-Squiggle." For years afterward, when I tried to explain to people just how deeply disturbing it was, I'd gather saliva at the back of my tongue and make a guttural *ccccchhhhh* sound, in and out, over and over. Just the vibration and swish of it in my ears would raise my blood pressure. If I made the sound for even a few seconds, David would turn away, shaking his head. It evoked late nights in the dark of Sammi's bedroom, holding her limp infant self on my lap while listening to the sound for hours and evenings after Ronni's bedtime when we had to turn up the volume on the television if we were holding Sammi. Even now, the thought of it makes me recoil.

But that fall after her first birthday, when she was hospitalized for the third time, something felt different. When I called Hilary from the hospital atrium one day after David arrived, she reminded me that her daughter, who had suffered through as many ear infections as Sammi, had never been hospitalized.

"You say 'it's only three days this time' like *any* days in the hospital are acceptable for a baby," she told me, her voice traveling across oceans and continents to bring me the perspective I lacked.

It was true that we'd been told she'd outgrow the wet, gurgling sound caused by that floppy tissue in her throat, but now we were past the arbitrary deadlines that Dr. Lynn and the pediatric ears, nose, and throat (ENT) doctor had set.

"She's too old for this, Mom," Dr. Lynn confirmed during our post-hospital checkup. "I want you to go back to that specialist and see what he thinks."

I really liked Dr. Holinger, the pediatric ENT. Aside from his sweet manner with Sammi, he was one of the only doctors we met in what would turn out to be years of hospital visits who bothered to learn my and David's names. Being called "Mom" by people who were not my children always bothered me. I'd tried a few times with other doctors— "Please, call me Debi"—but it never worked. Dr. Holinger, on the other hand, always looked us in the eye when he asked if we had any other questions.

The day after our visit with Dr. Lynn, I called the nurse who scheduled Dr. Holinger's appointments.

"Hello," I said into the phone, breastfeeding Sammi on my lap, "my daughter is a patient of Dr. Holinger's. She's just over twelve months old, has laryngomalacia, and just spent three days in the hospital with a cold. Her pediatrician wants Dr. Holinger to see her again."

"Does she have a tracheal tube?" asked the nurse.

"No," I said.

"Is she on supplemental oxygen?"

"No, they sent her home from the hospital without it," I answered, shifting Sammi to my shoulder to rub her back.

"Well, it doesn't sound like an emergency," droned the nurse. "I could get you an appointment in about eight weeks . . . excuse me. Can you hear me?"

"Yes, I can hear you fine." I moved Sammi to my other shoulder and swapped the phone to my other ear.

"Oh, I thought I heard static. Do you hear the static?"

"Oh," I said. "No. That's not static. That's my daughter. She's on my shoulder."

"That sound is the baby?" asked the nurse. "Is that her *breathing*?"

"Yes," I apologized. "Sorry. We call her Darth Baby. It's always like this after nursing when she has a cold."

"That sound is her *breathing*?" the nurse repeated.

In Dr. Holinger's office a week later, he raised his eyebrows when we told him that Sammi had suffered through at least ten ear infections that year.

"Of course, some of them might have been one ear infection that never really resolved," I said. "Sometimes she'd finish a round of antibiotics and then get another infection a day or so later."

Dr. Holinger nodded. "What about her eating?" he asked. "Does she like it?"

I almost laughed. When Hilary and her daughter Maya were visiting, I had been shocked by what Maya ate in a day. She was three months younger than Sammi and eating at least four times as much solid food. Sammi, on the other hand, was still stuck on halved blueberries, the dehydrated corn that melted in her mouth, and slivers of watermelon. She managed a few bites of jarred baby food at each meal. I told Dr. Holinger about all of this, and he pressed me for more.

"How about more solid foods? Does she like crackers?" he asked.

I shook my head. "No, it's pretty much just fruit and those corn kernels that melt."

He looked pensive for a moment, and then apologized as he turned back to his computer. After a few moments, he said, "Well, Debi, I think it's pretty clear that she needs ear tubes, and as long as we're going to put her under for that, I'd love to get a closer look at her airway. It's a very safe procedure and I do a lot of them. I just think it's time to see why she keeps getting so sick with these upper respiratory infections. I have some ideas, but let's just see how she looks and go from there."

Years later, a statement like that would have sent my antennae way up, crackling with a faint signal of danger. I would have pressed him to tell me what he was thinking, what "ideas" he had. I would have gone home and searched the internet for information about each possibility, joined some online support groups, and asked the members about their experiences with diagnosis. I would have gone into that ear tube and bronchoscopy day both more stressed and more prepared for the possibilities that awaited me.

Instead, being inexperienced, I went in with curiosity and low expectations. I'd been telling doctors and nurses that something further was wrong with Sammi for more than a year by then and had heard nothing but "overanxious mom" comments from everyone I asked. Becoming the prepared, expert mother of a medically complex child didn't happen overnight. I could pack a bag for the emergency room in fewer than five minutes that first year, but I was not in any way prepared for what was about to change in Sammi's—and my—life.

Within a few weeks of that meeting with Dr. Holinger, Sammi was in the operating room, where ear tubes were inserted and a long scope went down her trachea. All at once, in the somber gray waiting room at the hospital, we learned something that shone light on both the thirteen months that had passed and the next few months ahead of us. After the murkiness of the past year, the clarity was both an enormous relief and a painful punch to my gut.

Since David had visited his grandmother, who was suffering from pneumonia in another hospital, earlier that day, I'd brought my friend Cathy to keep me company during Sammi's procedure. It was supposed to be routine, and I'd promised Cathy we'd find somewhere fun to have lunch afterward. David and I thought that Dr. Holinger would tell us Sammi had a more serious case of gastrointestinal reflux, give us a more powerful prescription, and that would be that.

We were very, very wrong.

Instead of patting me patronizingly and sending us on our way, Dr. Holinger described to Cathy and me what he'd seen during the bronchoscopy he'd performed. It looked to him as though Sammi's aorta— the main artery coming out of her heart—had been malformed in the womb. It had, he thought, two equally spaced arches that had wrapped around her trachea and her esophagus. Sammi would need an operation to remove one of those arches, and they were sending someone from the cardiothoracic surgeon's office to talk with us in just a few minutes.

"You can take her home today," Dr. Holinger told me, "but no more solid food for her, OK? That esophagus is pretty tight."

"So just baby food, then?" I asked, fighting to speak through fear that felt like a hand gripping my lungs. "That's really all she eats most of the time anyway. Plus blueberries."

"No baby food, please," he said, "switch her to a liquid diet. She's still nursing, so you're in good shape on that."

I was indeed. After a year, Sammi was still nursing upward of eight or ten times a day. "Nurtch?" she'd say, pointing at my chest, and I'd scoop her into my arms and lower myself, cross-legged, to the nearest chair or couch or rug or patch of grass. My breasts belonged to her completely, and she knew it, patting them gently as her eyes fluttered closed.

In fact, just a little while later, Cathy and I found ourselves in a curtained-off area of the recovery suite, waiting as Sammi—still dopey from the anesthesia—nursed dreamily in my arms. My mind was racing from all of the information the advanced practice nurse had just shared: an operation as soon as possible, an incision down Sammi's shoulder blade, the word "ligate." I looked up at Cathy, tears in my eyes, and surveyed the room. "Where *am* I?" I asked her. Of course, I knew where I was, but I didn't understand, on a spiritual level, on a metaphysical level, how I'd come to be there. This sensation was repeated many times through the years, especially after effectively shutting off my emotions to get through another horror-filled moment in a hospital room or to receive yet another phone call with bad news. I'd take in the information, efficiently record it in my notebook or manage it as Sammi dozed in a hospital bed and then, a short time later, absorb the shock of it in my body and wonder what was *really* happening. The dream state I could invoke got me through the actual moment, but the emotions caught up to me, eventually, every time.

In the recovery room, behind the partition, Cathy looked me right in the eyes.

"You're feeding your baby," she said. "That's all you need to know right now."

We emerged from the hospital with a pile of paperwork—appointments to schedule and academic papers about the "double aortic arch" to read—and realized that we were ravenous. We walked across the street to the nearest bar and grill, where I ordered an enormous portabella mushroom sandwich with fries. We didn't talk much. When Sammi reached for a french fry (she loved to hold and gnaw on them), I didn't know what to do. Though I knew I shouldn't, I slit the side of the French fry open with a steak knife then used my spoon to scrape soft, greasy potato mush from it. I gathered up the mush and put it on the end of my finger, holding it out for Sammi, who licked it half-heartedly and pushed it away. In the end, I gave her a clean baby spoon from the diaper bag, and she sucked on that instead.

The weeks that followed were filled with fear. The instructions from the hospital were not to let her cry, lest her blood pressure go up and choke her from the inside. David and I took shifts, driving her to sleep all night long. Amid the unending exhaustion and anxiety and heightened awareness of the yellow lines down the center of the road during our 3:00 a.m. drives, I can picture only one source of calories for me: the child-size cup of Sprite I would get from the Burger King drive-through, open all night. Any bigger than that, and I'd have to contend with the need to pee.

The day of the surgery arrived, finally, and while my parents took care of Ronni, David and I took Sammi to the hospital in the dark, early morning. His mother, sister, and brother-in-law were there with us, waiting as anxiously as we were, making sure that, in my stupor, I remembered to eat something. I didn't know it at the time, but I would eat crispy hash brown patties in the basement cafeteria of the hospital dozens of times in the years to come.

Thankfully, the surgery went well. When we reunited with Sammi in her room in the cardiac ICU, she was attached to four different IVs— one in each arm and leg, every limb splinted so she wouldn't thrash the IVs out of place. She looked like she had been dropped from a great height onto her back, arms and legs splayed out around her, clothed in only a diaper. Thankfully, she was heavily drugged; she didn't react at all to our tentative kisses around the perimeter of the oxygen mask that covered her mouth and nose.

But as the nurse began to adjust her pain medication down later that night, she regained her sense of her one and only goal in the world: to nurse. Anytime I tried to hold her, she thrashed in my arms, desperate. We set her gently, gingerly, into David's lap, carefully winding all the tubing across his legs, a soft blanket covering her. She still fussed and seemed unsettled. We were like new parents, trying to figure out this unfamiliar version of our child who required special handling, who was addled by drugs and suddenly coughing and frightened by the sputum in her own mouth, the first time her airway had ever been open enough for a productive cough. We didn't know how to settle her.

Finally, I had a revelation. Reaching into my wallet, I removed a photo of Ronni. "Want to see Ronni?" I asked Sammi. "Want to hold her picture?"

"Rah-ree!" Sammi cried, hoarsely, her first word since morning. She grabbed the photo with the three fingers protruding from the IV splint and fell asleep holding it. When we carefully laid her back in the bed, I placed her baby doll, Raizl—the same type of doll as Ronni's beloved Shayna—next to her. Asleep, she clutched Raizl with the fingers of her other hand, and—for the first time in her life—she slept for nine consecutive hours.

The next morning, David and I were so absorbed in entertaining Sammi that we didn't notice Dr. Backer, the cardiothoracic surgeon, standing on the other side of the glass door.

He had a surprised look on his face as he watched us. Sammi continued to giggle and jab at a paper with her marker. We saw him say something to the nurse and wave feebly at Sammi. She looked up and used her marker to wave back at him.

At this, he cracked a smile and came into the room. "Look at you," he said to Sammi.

He explained that he'd be getting us out of the ICU as quickly as he could; Sammi didn't need that level of care anymore. "There are some really sick kids in here," he said. "She doesn't belong." He told us his nurse would see us before Sammi was released, which would probably be the next day.

"Good luck," he said. "She'll be a new little girl."

After only two nights in the hospital, it was over. She came home with stitches down the length of her shoulder blade, free to eat a "normal diet," whatever that was, but at her three-week postsurgical checkup, Dr. Lynn was not impressed with her recovery. Even after a gastroenterologist had dilated Sammi's esophagus in an outpatient procedure two weeks later, Sammi's eating hadn't improved for more than a day or two. She'd gone from a too-small sixteen-and-a-half pounds to a far-too-small sixteen pounds even.

"You've gotta get some pounds on her, Mom," she told me after scooping Sammi off the scale. "She can't lose any more ground or we're going to have to consider tube feedings."

She went on to suggest a variety of ways we could increase the number of calories Sammi ate, ranging from adding cream to her blueberries to giving her two cups of Carnation Instant Breakfast each day. What I wanted to say, but didn't, was that unless we could get the Carnation Instant Breakfast to come out of my breasts, Sammi wasn't going to drink it. Still, we did our best.

First, I began what would become my most time-consuming hobby over the next decade: online research. "High-calorie foods for babies" and "high-fat foods" and "baby gain weight" were searches repeated over and over, followed with experiments conducted in the high chair every day. After many false starts, we found a cup that Sammi could manage, an expensive one that we bought on a whim one day. We could never find another one, forcing us to protect the one we had with almost as much fierceness as we'd protect Sammi herself.

"Don't forget Sammi's cup," we said to each other every time we left the house. If we forgot the cup, she wouldn't drink a thing. As Dr. Lynn had suggested, we started filling it every day with Carnation Instant Breakfast, trying every flavor before landing on chocolate as the one she drank with the most enthusiasm. At fifteen months old but not even on the growth chart for her age, Sammi looked like a strange combination of a six-month-old baby and the toddler she was becoming. She sat in the baby seat at the grocery store holding her chocolate drink, while I inwardly cringed at the stares I imagined coming from all the other moms in the store. I was sure they were thinking *who gives a little baby chocolate milk?*

I'd felt that sense of being secretly judged before. In the weeks between our meeting with Dr. Holinger and the day he discovered her double aortic arch, he'd referred her for a few sessions of "feeding therapy," a specialty area of speech therapy that I didn't know existed. He'd wanted to be sure, I realized in retrospect, that Sammi's swallowing and eating issues were not behavioral. The feeding therapists suggested that I bring Sammi to her first appointment hungry so that they could observe her when she would be likely to eat a lot. At her late afternoon appointment, after having eaten exactly two bites of peaches and nursed several times throughout the day, she managed to eat three peas and a bite of watermelon, followed by a two-ounce bottle. The feeding therapists had clucked their tongues at me and declared Sammi far too dependent on nursing, and I felt shame heat my cheeks.

The first thing they had suggested was that I keep Sammi to a strict schedule of nursing and offering solid foods. She was "allowed" to nurse three times a day and was to be put in her high chair three times a day for her solid food meals and twice for small snacks. During those solid food meals, she was to be removed from her chair after thirty minutes regardless of how much or little she had eaten. Snacks were allotted fifteen minutes.

This plan did not resonate with me. It was the polar opposite of my philosophy of feeding children according to their appetite. Nursing both Sammi and Ronni had been incredibly rewarding. To hold my baby quietly in my arms, snuggle her close, smell her skin as she grew warm and soft, feel her body relax, and sense the safety and comfort that she felt intertwine with the experience of eating: this was one of the few completely enjoyable experiences of mothering babies for me. It was also everything I think a baby deserves: undivided attention, nourishment of body and soul, and loving touch. The clinical schedule prescribed by the feeding therapists was downright cruel in contrast.

A week later, we visited them again. I told them frankly that the week had been hell, mostly because I was fighting my instincts. The only thing that I felt had helped was switching her one bottle a day to the slower-flowing nipple, which resulted in less gasping and pulling away. We weighed her, and after this one week of dictating exactly when and for how long Sammi was allowed to eat, she had lost half a pound. If she had a feeding disorder—or even if she was just plain "picky"—she wouldn't have refused to eat even the solid foods she liked all week.

The therapist said that I could go back to nursing her when I wanted to for now, with an eye to increasing her solids intake slowly, as long as she continued to grow and gain weight. Looking across the low therapy table where Sammi sat listlessly poking at her watermelon pieces, the therapist leaned closer and whispered, "Sometimes, that mommy instinct is right on target."

After we'd identified the structural problem that had constricted her esophagus and she'd had the surgery to repair it, I realized that if I was going to keep her off a feeding tube—and damn it, I *was* going to keep her off a feeding tube—I had to let go of all the notions I had about appropriate diet. This was about calories in, pounds on, period. With that as my baseline requirement, adjusting for her preferences, I was going to have to find fatty foods that were soft. Just before the specialist had diagnosed her, she'd tried grains again and hadn't repeated the vomiting, so we were without dietary restrictions. What foods were out there that might appeal to my strange, appetite-free baby girl?

We started with avocado, which was a mild success; if it was mashed, she'd get her fingers messy with it and suck it off of them, but not in the kind of quantity that would constitute a meal. I'd never liked avocados myself, so I never knew how to buy them. Sometimes they were too soft and brown; sometimes hard and crunchy and impossible to mash. If she ate two bites, the rest would turn brown and unappetizing, and the expense of buying these fussy little green footballs made me anxious.

Next, we tried whole cream. I poured half an inch into one of Sammi's small plastic bowls then added blueberries. I tried mixing them in the cream to coat them but then watched dejectedly as the cream beaded up and slid off the berries. Undeterred, I'd do this several times a day, since Sammi was willing to eat them. I'd watch anxiously as the occasional droplet of cream made it into Sammi's mouth, mentally tallying it up: had she eaten about two teaspoons of cream today? At fifty-two calories per tablespoon, it wasn't much, but it was better than plain blueberries at five calories per tablespoon. I counted bites of avocado, licks of refried beans, droplets of cream. It was never enough.

One night at dinner, David was putting Brummel & Brown margarine—a yogurt-based spread—on crackers. To our surprise, Sammi reached for one, and when David held it for her to take a bite, she licked the margarine off and pushed the cracker away. He put more margarine on, and she did it again.

"I have an idea," he said, and went into the kitchen, returning with one of her baby spoons. He put the soggy cracker back on his plate and dipped the spoon in the tub of margarine.

"Oh my gosh," I said, "you're not . . ."

But before I could complete my sentence, he'd fed Sammi a spoonful of margarine—and she'd eaten it. "Hey, it's calories, right?" he said in a singsong voice as he gave her another bite. I excused myself, locked myself in the bathroom, and gagged.

And then I discovered extra virgin coconut oil.

At room temperature, extra virgin coconut oil is the consistency of petroleum jelly. It's thick and viscous, a translucent white that shines in the light. I'd never seen it before the day that I googled "most fattening vegetarian ingredient" and saw that it had 116 calories per tablespoon and—even better—almost no flavor at all. With any heat applied to it, it melted into a thin oil that disappeared into whatever else was in the bowl. It was a stealth food. I bought some immediately.

First I tried adding it to the stage-one jarred infant food Sammi still liked, mostly sweet potatoes and, of course, blueberries, but it didn't mix well unless the food was warm. I tried warming a ramekin of the oil and drizzling it into the baby food, but that only worked when we first opened a jar. She never finished a whole jar in one sitting, so then I had to microwave the half-full jar to melt the oil, more than once burning my fingers. Plus, she never ate enough to make it worth the effort of cajoling her and sneaking food into her mouth, a high-stakes experience for me that left us both anxious. I didn't want to force-feed her. I needed a better delivery system, something she loved and could even feed herself.

My next attempt was to warm a bowl of blueberries just enough to melt the coconut oil. As I mixed them in the bowl, I spooned a little powdered sugar onto them, which helped the oil stick to the berries. This, finally, was an effective way to deliver calories into Sammi's tiny body. She sat happily pinching berries between her fingers and stuffing them into her mouth. With a full set of teeth now, she chewed them to a messy pulp that smeared across her cheeks in greasy purple swipes. I gave her ten berries at a time, and sometimes she asked for more by holding the empty bowl and shaking it until lavender-colored oil flecked her hair.

By December, she had gained half a pound, finally reaching her presurgery weight. Dr. Lynn applauded my efforts, though she grimaced at my triumphant description of the blueberries.

"How about some protein, Mom?" she asked me. "Can you get her to eat beans? I know you're one of those vegetarians."

Dr. Lynn never approved of our vegetarianism, though she rarely talked about it. Those moments when we were desperate for better ways to feed Sammi—and there would be more as time went on—inspired her worry.

I'd been a vegetarian since I was fourteen. Looking down one day at my mother's chicken soup, I suddenly became aware that, in effect, I was spooning bird juice into my mouth. It happened all at once—a horrible realization that made me retch. In the days that followed, I begged my parents to let me stop eating meat. At first, they agreed to a two-week trial, during which I made myself a cheese or peanut butter sandwich when dinner was going to be meat, and then, when it was clear that I was done for good, they began adding more vegetarian options to our regular diet. In college, I subsisted on bagels with swiss cheese, ramen noodles, and macaroni and cheese, splurging twice a month on the $4 veggie burgers sold at the student union, the only place on campus that sold such a thing in the early 1990s.

David is not a vegetarian, but his family's history of heart disease is significant. When we were first married, I learned how to step out of my body briefly so I could gingerly spear a raw chicken breast and drop it into a casserole dish to cook for him, but after his own cholesterol started to climb in his early thirties, he agreed to eat vegetarian food at home, with rare exceptions when he grilled outside. We'd decided to raise both children as vegetarians until they were old enough to ask for meat themselves. When Sammi was creeping her way up from sixteen and a half pounds that first winter after her surgery, Dr. Lynn was subtly suggesting that meat would be the best way to help her gain weight.

I couldn't bring myself to do it, though. Sammi had yet to eat anything thicker than refried beans; I doubted very much that she would go for chicken nuggets. Still, one day I took a deep breath and bought a jar of chicken and rice baby food. I gave it to David that night when he came home from work and then left the room when he sat down across from Sammi's high chair to feed it to her. I couldn't even watch; I went upstairs to the bathroom attached to our bedroom, turned on the water in the sink, and sat on the floor for ten minutes, half-reading a book. When I felt enough time had elapsed, I went downstairs.

Sammi was sitting in her high chair eating blueberries. I looked pointedly at David, raising my eyebrows.

"Nope," he said, gesturing at the jar of food. "She's not into it."

I knew the rule about offering a baby a food ten times before deciding for certain that she doesn't like it, but Sammi had loved blueberries at first bite. I wasn't going to try chicken and rice ten times. I needed to come up with my own way to feed her.

The one food with protein that Sammi had been willing to eat so far was refried beans. The rest of us weren't that into beans, in general— David really didn't like them—but maybe there was some other way to make them for Sammi. Years before, I'd had that subscription to *Vegetarian Times*. The recipes I'd clipped were still half-sorted in my little black binder; I pulled it out and sifted through them, noting anything that seemed like a good fit for Sammi.

The recipe I tried first was a simple one that I made even simpler. It was called, no frills required, "Chickpea Soup." The recipe described it as a "centerpiece unto itself," but after making at least a hundred pots of this soup, I can imagine this only as the centerpiece of a very simple peasant meal, the kind of meal that was all I could bring myself to prepare in 2006 when I made this soup for the first time and unwittingly saved Sammi from a feeding tube.

The ingredient list was short—just eight ingredients—and I immediately cut it to seven, several improvised. I learned to keep these ingredients in the house at all times. When the container of "Sammi's soup" in the fridge was down to a cup or less, I quickly made another batch, starting with the combination that birthed almost every soup I would love from that point on: olive oil and a chopped onion.

Of course, sometimes I had only vegetable oil, and that was OK then. I didn't really know the difference between kinds of oil in 2006— an unimaginable thought even just five years later—but then, I shrugged and measured one tablespoon of oil. One carefully diced onion sizzled as it hit the bottom of a pot my mother had given me during my first bridal shower, a dented and battered pot that came to America on the boat with her great-grandmother. I invoked my ancestors more than once while making soup in this pot: *please, help me feed my baby.*

Next went in two cans of chickpeas, whatever brand was cheapest. Years later I would feel guilty, recalling the liquid around the chickpeas that went down the drain, which I learned was called aquafaba and could be whipped with sugar in my stand mixer to make meringue. But when Sammi was a baby I needed to feed, I rinsed the chickpeas of this liquid until the water ran clear. They dropped onto the browned onions and oil and sizzled until I used a yellowed plastic mixing spoon to combine them.

Finally, a haphazard toss of a bay leaf—for which I'd searched, that first time in the grocery store, through the lettuces and plastic clamshells of dill before a store employee guided me to the dry spice aisle—and half a cup of chopped parsley, a teaspoon and a half of salt, and four cups of water. The lemon juice at the end of the recipe was far too much work, so I omitted it. Within ten minutes, the soup would be boiling, suffusing the house with the peppery smell of bay leaf.

"Sammi's soup?" David would ask when he came home from work, sniffing the air.

The first time I'd tried to feed it to her had been a holy, mystical experience. The last step in the recipe, after it had cooked down and the chickpeas were plump and sensual in their bath, was to puree the entire endeavor, minus the bay leaf, which I'd chased around the pot, stabbing at it with a pair of tongs. Bringing the immersion blender out after its failure in my efforts to feed Sammi homemade pureed baby food months before gave me a surprising pang of post-traumatic distress. *This is stupid*, I heard myself say as I lowered it into the pot. *She'll never eat it.*

But she did.

The soup was a golden color, the beige of the chickpeas against the flecks of parsley and the shine of the olive oil. I cooled it to just warm, put some in Sammi's little pink plastic bowl, and sat down across from her to await her rejection of it. At seventeen months old, her reddish infant hair was gone and replaced with a surprising tuft of blond. She had teeth on top and bottom, and her dark brown eyes with long lashes forever reminded me of my mother's laughing ones. Though she had regained her presurgery weight, she had grown taller without gaining any more, and that day, her eyes peered at me from under a forehead whose skull bones protruded at the hairline, skin so fair that I could see the blue veins crossing her cheek.

"It's yummy soup," I said, brandishing a spoon coated in soft rubber.

She opened her mouth for me—not a given, even at mealtime—and I put a tiny spoonful of the soup in her mouth. I watched as she sucked in her cheeks and tapped the tip of her tongue on the edge of her lips. She swallowed. Then she put her fingertips on the edge of the bowl, looked me in the eye, and opened her mouth again.

She ate the whole serving. Admittedly, I'd learned over many months of wasting food not to fill the bowl much, but the number of times that I scraped the bottom to get to the last morsels were few if not zero. I felt a panic rise in me. *Why hadn't I filled the bowl fuller? Should I let her hold the bowl and fill another? Will she eat this soup out of another bowl? If I take this bowl away now to refill it, she may lose interest. Was it the soup or just luck?*

I took a risk and said, "Want some more?"

She made a shouting noise. I stood up and refilled the bowl. This time, she ate half of it before pursing her lips closed and shaking her head. It was the most I'd seen her eat at one sitting in her entire life.

From then on, I took the soup out of the pot when it was boiling hot, added a few tablespoons of extra virgin coconut oil, and swirled it through until it melted and disappeared into the puree. Then I left it to cool before feeding it to Sammi, adding one or two hundred extra calories to her favorite meal.

Over the years, I would learn to adapt this soup in nearly a dozen ways. When we began subscribing to a weekly vegetable share from a farm, I substituted the parsley for any cooking green we'd receive, from spinach to beet greens to kale. I substituted the water for vegetable consommé, adding more flavor. I left out the bay leaf if I didn't have one. I made it without oil and chickpeas when Sammi had to be on a fat-free diet at age eight, substituting lentils and softening the onions in broth. I froze quarts of it, brought pots of it to sick friends, and finally, one day when Sammi was thirteen, I taught her to make it herself.

"It's good!" she told me, standing with one hand under the spoon, blowing gently. "It smells like my chickpea soup."

"It's the first thing I really learned to cook for you," I answered, leaning down to taste it from the spoon.

"Really?" Her eyes got wider. "You didn't learn this from your mom?"

I shook my head and squeezed her around the shoulders, catching a tuft of the hair she'd dyed pink earlier that year. "Nope, I found this recipe in a magazine."

"It tastes like *your* food," she said, dropping the spoon in the sink and turning off the heat under the pot. "It doesn't taste like a magazine recipe."

By then, she was right, in a way. I'd memorized that recipe, internalized it, rubbed its essence into what it meant to be Sammi's mother. The very DNA of our home carried in it the scent and aura of chickpea soup and all of the other foods that I learned to cook over the years. Just like the taste of tapioca custard would always be the taste of my childhood home, my ultimate comfort food imprinted with memories of my mother, Sammi would never taste this food without some subconscious neuron firing into her memory of my face, staring at hers hopefully, a spoonful of her savior in my hand.

4

TOSTADAS, A REVELATION

After my success with the chickpea soup, I felt empowered to try other things. It had become clear to me during my many internet searches that simple articles on "tips for feeding picky toddlers" would not meet the needs of my family. We were contending with my own lactose intolerance, our shared vegetarianism, Sammi's refusal to eat almost everything that wasn't soft, and, at the same time, my desperation not to quash Ronni's voracious appetite and willingness to try new things by forcing her to subsist on a diet of soup and fruit and the frozen macaroni and cheese she liked. I wanted to be better at feeding *all* of us.

Shortly after Ronni turned five and just before Sammi turned two, we moved from our townhouse in the city of Chicago just a few miles north to Evanston, a nearby suburb. Our new kitchen was located in the corner of the L-shaped first floor; within a few steps I could see into the sunny dining room and the cozy living room. If I stood on my toes, I could see over the counter to the child-sized wooden table where the girls perched on little chairs to eat breakfast, color, and chatter with each other. It was the perfect layout for me to settle in and build a kitchen repertoire.

But one thing was missing, I would realize in short order: I had no one to teach me how to cook. So many of the foods my family would come to love over the years were either other people's recipes or inspired by them. When we first moved to Evanston, though, I didn't know anyone. My mother, who was a very good cook, moved with my father to retire clear across the country only a few months after we bought our house, and although there were recipes emailed back and forth and holiday visits that included a lot of cooking together, what I needed most were other parents of children close in age to mine, or even a little bit older, to share the kind of cooking and baking lore that travels so well between families.

Instead, it was just me and the girls most of the time for many months. Because Sammi's pediatrician and the otolaryngologist had told us to keep her away from other children and their germs after her hospitalizations due to simple colds, I didn't even really know many other parents, let alone other parents near where I lived. Once again, the internet became my best resource, along with a few cookbooks I'd begun to acquire, especially the one that came with my new subscription to the CSA produce box I received twenty weeks a year. My cooking was still very simple, but I found that I was learning some basic skills just by noticing patterns. Soups started with fat and onions; baked goods started by combining wet ingredients with wet and dry ingredients with dry; greens cooked down to nothing but root vegetables held their volume. It seems obvious now, but these are the things we learn cooking at the elbows of our mothers, and I'd never taken the time to learn from mine when she was still nearby.

In August 2007, though, a generational transfer of culinary learning took place in the most unlikely way: I got a recipe from my paternal grandmother Dorothy, who had died when my father was only twelve. One afternoon, my father received a call from his cousin, who was cleaning out some drawers in his aunt's house. In a pile of other papers, she found two handwritten recipe cards labeled with my grandmother's name. More than fifty years old by then, those recipes had somehow survived intact. My father's cousin sent the recipes to him right away, and he sent them to me. Both were recipes for Ashkenazi Jewish noodle puddings, known as *lokshen kugels*. The kugels I knew as a child were all sweet lokshen kugels; my mother's recipe had cottage cheese and sugar and sometimes sliced peaches or apples in it.

But these kugels from my grandmother were both very different. One was a pecan-and-brown-sugar kugel made in a ring pan; I discounted it immediately because it contained cottage cheese, something I couldn't easily replace with a nondairy option. The other one, though, contained cream cheese, for which I did have a reasonable dairy-free analogue. I thought it was worth a try.

The recipe contained egg noodles, cream cheese, butter, and sugar—so far, pretty traditional—but it also contained apricot nectar, which was unusual. I searched the grocery store with the girls strapped into the seat at the front of the cart, steering us up and down the aisles until I reached the Mexican section. There, cans that looked like they were meant for soda held nectars of peach, mango, guava, and—finally!—apricot. They each had one ounce more than the recipe required, and for years I was so afraid of changing one more thing that I painstakingly measured it to omit one ounce. By the time this kugel became famous in my own community—even gracing the tables at Ronni's bat mitzvah eight years later—I'd stopped bothering to leave out that last ounce. Recipes, I would come to learn, can evolve much like folk songs, with a lyric or an ounce of nectar changed here and there, the common ancestor still nodding in agreement and holding it all together despite the changes.

That first time, though, I followed the recipe to the letter with the exception of my nondairy cream cheese and margarine. It was outrageously good, creamy and sweet, the bite of the noodles just right under a crust of sugared cornflake topping. Ronni, who had vowed that no kugel would ever be as good as David's Aunt Maxine's kugel (which used pineapple), took one bite and closed her eyes in delight.

"Whose kugel is this?" she asked me, digging into another bite.

"It's my grandma's," I said, smiling.

"Buba?" Ronni asked, referring to my mother's mother.

"No," I answered, "Zayda's mom, my grandma Dorothy." Then I told her the story of his cousin finding the recipe, and her eyes got wider and brighter, and she said we had to always call this "Grandma Dorothy's Kugel."

I began to take this kugel everywhere, the first really successful recipe that I could make for other people. I took a picture of the kugel with my hand holding my grandma's picture over it, whispered, "thanks, grandma," and felt a little bit more capable in the kitchen. Perhaps because it came directly from my own lineage, the literal food of my ancestors, I felt a connection to it that gave me enough confidence to continue. From kugel, I moved to matzo ball soup, guided by instinct that told me to make the matzo balls themselves from a mix. The soup, though, I made from scratch, tasting and trying and learning, calling my mom to ask how she cooked a whole onion in the pot, how *much* dill she sprinkled on top, how much garlic, how many carrots.

"I don't know, a few cloves?" she'd answer. "Not too much, though. How big a pot?"

Years later, I would stand Ronni and then Sammi at the stove and show them how to trim the top and bottom of the onion, to run a blade along the one side gently just to split the outer skin and peel it off, to drop the peeled onion whole in the pot and ensure the water covered it. I would teach them to roll chilled matzo ball batter between wet hands so it didn't stick, to cover the pot and not peek inside. They would beg me to leave out the dill. Whenever Sammi was at her most miserable, a pot of matzo ball soup would lift her chin into the air, her curious nose sniffing, and then an audible sigh would release itself from her mouth as she exhaled. "Matzo ball soup?" she'd ask with anticipation, though, of course, she'd known.

The third in the triad of Ashkenazi triumphs in my new kitchen came two days before my brother's wedding. I'd offered to host a Sabbath dinner on Friday night, inviting his future mother-in-law and father-in-law, sisters-in-law, and brother-in-law, along with our own parents. My mother and father came to help me cook. I'd planned one of the few dishes I made well—vegetable potpie—and my mother promised to make chicken. We had a stack of printed-out salad recipes, a chocolate chip cake recipe my mother had made a thousand times, and a plan to make a traditional braided egg bread—challah—based on a recipe my friend Hilary had sent me.

Hilary lived in Israel with her husband and her daughter who was the same age as Sammi. She'd go on to have three more children—all boys—but then, it was just her and Maya and her husband Eytan. In an instant message conversation a few months back, she'd described hoisting Maya onto a stool at the counter to pound the dough and told me how much they loved having fresh bread every week. The image in my head was idyllic, and I'd decided that Hilary's challah had to be the one we made. She emailed me the recipe, and I printed it and set it aside. My mother had made challah often when I was a child, but I remembered it as a little drier than I liked. Hilary had told me hers was chewy and soft. I was ready.

That Friday morning, my mother and I made the potpie and got the chicken ready; we prepped the salads and baked the chocolate cake. At one in the afternoon, we pulled out the challah recipe, planning for the two risings so that the challah itself would still be warm out of the oven at dinnertime. As we started assembling the ingredients and mixing them, my mother frowned and held the recipe up.

"How many eggs?" she asked.

I took the paper from her and looked again. There were none listed. Challah, after all, was egg bread—how could we make it without the eggs? I tried reaching Hilary in all the ways we usually communicated—email, Facebook Messenger, even a long-ignored app we'd used when she was traveling with little access to internet. No response. It was nearly ten at night in Israel, and she was pregnant with her second child and probably fast asleep. My mother looked at the recipe, at the contents of the bowl on the counter, and seemed to count in her head.

"Let's use three eggs," she said, finally. "What's the worst thing that could happen? We can always run out and buy a challah."

Cautiously, we added the eggs and kneaded the dough. After a while, it resembled the challah dough I'd seen my mother make before, including the dough in a beloved family video of me, my mother, and her mother making it together when I was only four. In the video, I stood on a stool, my long braids tied in loops at the back of my neck, singing a song about making challah that I'd learned in preschool. During the intervening years since that video had been made, I couldn't remember ever making it again, but here I was in my own kitchen, thirty years later, learning how to eyeball the right number of eggs, my own daughter giggling and playing in the next room while her sister was in school. The challahs came out perfectly, and when I caught up with Hilary online the next week, she told me she never put eggs in hers. In my expectations about what constituted a proper loaf, I'd done a little folk-music treatment on the recipe. Like my grandmother's kugel, Hilary's challah wasn't completely loyal to the original recipe, but—in the opinion of everyone who tasted it—it was fantastic.

I got braver, searching for more recipes I could expand, contract, and edit. Next came soups and stews: another chickpea soup recipe, this one flavored with tomatoes and half a dozen Indian spices from which I omitted the fresh mint and added steamed broccoli, and a Greek lentil stew with only a handful of ingredients to which I added stewed tomatoes and vinegar. Both of these I associated with my new friend Clare, the mother of one of Ronni's best friends. I met Clare soon after moving to Evanston, and our daughters' instant friendship spawned ours, too. Though Clare didn't enjoy cooking the way I did, we had complementary skills and—more importantly—an abiding love for eating communally. After school, we often combined households during the late afternoon to let the kids play together in one of our yards while we chatted. Eventually, the children would tire of the clementines or pretzels we were feeding them, and we'd shrug and scrounge for what, between our pantries, we could combine for a meal. Sometimes it was the lentil stew that her daughter Zora loved; the potatoes and hard-boiled eggs with dill sauce Clare had learned to make in the Czech Republic; or a half-hearted "fro-za" (frozen pizza). Other times, I spread hummus on bagels and topped them with tomatoes and cucumbers, or made pasta with shredded parmesan and steamed broccoli, or warmed up some leftover kugel. It was wonderful to share the kitchen duties with Clare, her quiet industriousness making light work of the dishes.

But the Indian-spiced chickpea soup I discovered in an unused cookbook that first winter was the best of all. After I made it the first time, I knew it would be my new standby. Full of whole chickpeas, cubed potatoes and carrots, diced celery, and onions, it simmered in a broth with tomatoes and all kinds of warm spices—ginger, cardamom, turmeric, garam masala—until its smell alone seemed to warm me. Adding the broccoli at the end had been a casual, last-minute decision, a bowl leftover in my fridge that needed to be eaten. It made the soup even better, adding texture and chew. The day after I made it the first time, Clare was lounging on my couch, watching our kids play, when she asked if I had anything warm to eat. I gave her a mug of it, and the ecstasy on her face after the first bite had me utterly hooked.

I loved feeding people. Of course, I'd known how rewarding it was to feed Ronni as a baby and how much fun it was to share my grandmother's kugel, but this was something else. There was a need that I had fulfilled; what's more, Clare loved the soup so much that she asked for the recipe. Even better, she filled a quart-sized mason jar with it a few months later and took it when she visited her mother, who was sick with the flu. It became a food with a history then. Saying "I'm making the spiced chickpea soup" was shorthand between us for something like "I'm feeling a need to be warm, nourished, and feel accomplished; I gathered the ingredients for this delicious food we both love, and now we'll both get a moment of enjoyment out of remembering how it tastes and feels."

All that pleasure I'd begun to feel when feeding people, though, disappeared into a black hole when it came to feeding Sammi. At two years old, she was still impossibly small and still shockingly hard to feed. She still carried what felt like my personal badge of shame into every doctor's appointment: a note on her chart that stated, accusingly, "failure to thrive," which I read as "failure to feed." By age two, she hadn't even reached the average weight of a one-year-old, and though she was willing to try a lot of different foods now, she seldom ate enough to qualify as a meal. She gobbled up anything soft and wet like berries or melon or chopped cucumbers; she ate her chickpea soup and small amounts of macaroni and cheese, but her other eating habits were only getting stranger.

"Spicy pickles!" she'd call out gleefully when the sharp Israeli pickles came out of the can. She'd eat two or three of them, an otherwise unheard-of amount of food for her, but the next day, she'd somehow survive on half a tiny bowl of cereal and a handful of raspberries until dinner. She'd say yes when I offered yogurt with berries—I called it "berried treasure"—but mostly picked out the fruit, saying she didn't like yogurt.

"Then why did you say you wanted it?" I'd ask, frustrated.

"I didn't *want* yogurt," she'd respond, sliding off her chair to run away and play.

Dr. Lynn thought that this was because—to my surprise as much as anyone else's—she was still breastfeeding. During the first year of her life, it was all that sustained her, and during the second year, it probably provided at least half of her daily calories. I was terrified of taking it away from her—and, frankly, away from me. It wasn't that I enjoyed the act of nursing her much anymore; she was talking and walking and sometimes climbing while she nursed, pulling at me as I sat in a chair and seethed. It wasn't even that I thought I had to anymore; I believed Dr. Lynn when she said that Sammi was choosing not to eat because she didn't have to, as long as she could nurse. I kept nursing her because something in my head just kept telling me it wasn't time yet.

I couldn't explain it. My mother's instinct had reared its head before and been right. When Sammi's months of sleep training had driven me almost to the brink of hysteria myself, I'd been told all parents hate sleep training. After Sammi's cardiac surgery, I'd learned all that crying was likely terribly painful for her, as increased blood pressure in her aorta squeezed her airway and esophagus even tighter. When I'd raced into the emergency room, holding my gasping and wheezing three-, four-, and twelve-month-old baby in my arms, I'd insisted it had to be something more than just a respiratory infection—and then the specialist had found her double aortic arch. I was learning to trust my instincts when it came to Sammi, and in her third year, I was trusting that same instinct in every way that related to feeding her. It wasn't until she was almost three years old that I succumbed to the pressure to wean her.

By the time she turned four, we'd had even more medical drama in the form of badly infected adenoids and tonsils that had to be removed, but by then, my prowess in the kitchen had begun to expand even more. She ate popsicles and cold butternut squash soup, turning her nose up at the tapioca custard I'd made from my mother's recipe. But even though the doctor had told us *this* would be the thing that finally helped her to eat enough to grow at an appropriate pace, it didn't. During the surgery, the doctor had noticed acid damage to her esophagus from acid reflux and continued compression on her airway from the damage done by the double aortic arch before it was repaired.

"She'll grow out of them, Mom," Dr. Lynn told me. "Just hang in there."

By the middle of her fourth year, we'd simply accepted that she was a poor eater. There was no magic moment after the cardiac surgery or the tonsil/adenoid surgery when she suddenly developed a bigger appetite or had a growth spurt, and despite the doctors' promises to the contrary, I wasn't surprised. All her favorite foods were still fruits and pickles, olives and soups. She would taste anything but seldom eat more than a few bites, and the things she refused were all dense or dry (bread, tofu, cookies) or thick and heavy (yogurt, cream sauces, milkshakes). It wasn't possible to grow a child on strawberries, and I knew it. Every bit of pressure I got from her doctors about trying meat or asking her to drink more Carnation Instant Breakfast sounded as ridiculous to me as asking her to eat bricks. I knew it the way I knew the feel of her soft cheek on mine; she could not eat those things.

By the spring before her fifth birthday, she'd begun gagging and coughing regularly. I'd heard her do it before, of course, an older-child version of her raspy breathing as a baby. I'd hear a sickening kind of *urp* sound, and then she'd cough so hard her eyes watered. When I asked her what was wrong, she'd just shrug.

"It's just my cereal in my mouth," she'd say, an hour after breakfast, or "it's just my yogurt," half an hour after lunch.

Was her reflux worsening as she got older instead of getting better? I asked other parents I knew whose children had reflux as babies if this was true for them. All their kids had outgrown it. We'd kept Sammi from all the usual reflux triggers like lemon, chocolate, and tomatoes (with special dispensation from the pediatrician for Carnation Instant Breakfast). When I took her to see Dr. Lynn, she thought it was time to go back to the specialists at the children's hospital for another look.

It was a good thing I'd learned to cook. Sammi had an endoscopy— a procedure under general anesthesia in which a doctor expands the esophagus with air and examines it with cameras and lights. While her esophagus was stretched open, the gastroenterologist had taken a biopsy. The results were conclusive: Sammi's esophagus was covered in several spots with furrows, ridges, and patches of white blood cells called eosinophils.

The diagnosis the doctor made was a disease called *eosinophilic esophagitis*, an autoimmune condition in which the esophagus is coated with—and damaged by—these eosinophils, usually in response to a sensitivity to one or more food proteins. It's poorly understood even now, and it was understood even less back then, only ten years after it had been recognized as a disease. Sammi's care was transferred to the only specialist in eosinophilic esophagitis—also known as EoE—in the practice, who began by putting her on an elimination diet.

To begin, I immediately would remove dairy, soy, eggs, peanuts, tree nuts, and wheat from Sammi's already vegetarian diet. After six weeks, she would have another endoscopy and biopsy to see if the inflammation and presence of eosinophils had gone away. If they had, we'd choose one of those foods to add back to her diet. Then we would wait another six weeks while she ate that food and do another endoscopy. This would repeat with all of those foods until we found all of the foods that her body saw as adversarial. It could be just one food, or three, or all of them, or it could be that the food affecting her was not one of those common allergens and instead was something we couldn't predict. If that was the case, we'd have to consider either removing corn from her diet and trying again or giving up and attempting one of the other options: strong drugs or the elimination of all food from her diet, to be replaced by an unabashedly foul-tasting prescription formula, possibly given through a feeding tube.

To say that I was floored by the elimination of two-thirds of our diet just as I was beginning to love cooking is an understatement. David and I had decided we would not eat differently from Sammi when we were together; not for the first time in her life, Sammi's health challenges would guide our mealtimes. The first thing I had to do was look in our cabinets and figure out what in the world we were going to eat. Everything seemed to be marked with a red circle and a diagonal line: *no.* No to pasta. No to Sammi's favorite macaroni and cheese in a box. No to soy milk, the only milk she ever drank. No to tofu, no to seitan, no to fake chicken nuggets. No to almost every cereal she liked. No to pizza. No, no, no—everything in my cabinets suddenly looked like poison.

I sat on my kitchen floor while Ronni and Sammi—ages four and seven—were at day camp and preschool just blocks away, and I wept. How would I feed her?

As a child, I had experienced food as charged with all kinds of emotional value. I had memories of my mother's continual self-deprivation, her mantra humming in my teenaged ears like background music: *I'm not having any; I'm being good.* I'd gone through phases when I associated food with weakness and assigned every food a score based on some imaginary scale that took into account my level of activity that day, my desire to change my body, and my willpower. In trying to raise my own daughters differently, I'd fought hard for the right to eat according to internal body cues and desires, despite Sammi's seemingly nonexistent appetite. How could this way of living stand up to the path we were about to take?

On the day that I cradled my head in my hands on the kitchen floor after Sammi's diagnosis, I saw all that effort endangered. I didn't know how I could maintain my "all food is good food for different reasons" attitude while saying no to so many things. I lay there on the floor and stared at the opened cabinets above me, half-wishing they'd simply peel away from the wall and crush me beneath them so that I would not have to solve this problem on my own.

That moment, I saw the can of chickpeas on one of the pull-out drawers of my pantry cabinet. Chickpeas are actually OK, I thought. Without giving myself time to think, I turned to a fresh page in the notebook I'd started for this diet and wrote "yes" at the top of the page and then "chickpeas" on the first line.

I stood up and pulled out the drawer. Almost all the food in cans, I realized, would be fine for Sammi. I started writing things down:

> Tomatoes
> Black beans
> Cannellini beans
> Vegetable broth
> Olives
> Pumpkin
> Artichoke hearts

I removed the cans of Chinese seitan—made entirely of wheat—and put them in a box on the counter behind me. That became the "Land of No" that week, but for the moment, I turned my back on it and faced the cabinet again. I pulled out the top drawer where all my spices lived, and added to the list:

> All the spices!
> Olive oil
> Vegetable oil

Immediately, I knew how I would tell Ronni and Sammi what was about to happen. I wrote furiously as I cataloged the list of "yes" foods.

> Fruity Pebbles
> Cocoa Pebbles
> Dum-Dums lollipops
> Smarties candy

I opened the baking cabinet, the hardest part. Almost everything went behind me into the Land of No, but there were still a few things left behind:

Cornstarch
Baking powder
Baking soda
Powdered sugar
Regular sugar
Corn syrup
Tapioca
Jello
Cocoa powder
Vanilla extract
Peppermint extract
Lemon extract
Tahini

Further to the left, another cabinet door revealed staples I'd forgotten about:

White rice
Brown rice
Dried beans
Lentils
Oats
Oat bran
Pappadums

More things went to the Land of No, but my pantry was far from empty. In the fridge, I compartmentalized each shelf into *yes* and *no*, moving fruits and vegetables to one side and milk, cheese, and eggs to the other. I wrote in my notebook:

All the vegetables!
All the fruits!

And further down, for the benefit of the children, I added the details of their own favorites:

Bananas
Strawberries
Raspberries
Blueberries
Cantaloupe
Watermelon
Apples
Pears
Mangos
Peaches
Nectarines
Pineapple
Plums
Apricots
Broccoli
Peas
Corn
Spinach
Arugula
Basil
Carrots
Sweet potatoes
Potatoes
Beets
Butternut squash
Green beans
Asparagus

There was food left in the house, after all, and I hadn't even gone to the grocery store to investigate alternatives. That night, we broke the news to Ronni and Sammi, taking turns reading from the list of "yes" foods. I snuck Ronni back downstairs after we'd taken Sammi to bed and talked to her about the secret box of snacks I planned to keep hidden away for her to take to school in the fall so she didn't have to eat the same thing Sammi ate and promised we'd make plans for her to go to friends' houses to eat pizza and noodles there.

I spent days and days after that trying to craft meals that looked at least a little familiar and to learn techniques for baking vegan, gluten free, and nut free. I learned from my friend Christine how to make basmati rice without measuring anything; my mother-in-law and sister-in-law showed up at my house with bag after bag of discoveries from their local health food stores; and a friend of a friend with celiac disease told me about the latest allergen-free baking mixes. But the food that made the biggest difference again came from my history.

More than five years before, I'd organized a mother-blessing ceremony, also known sometimes as a blessingway ceremony, for one of my closest friends. Andrea, my neighbor across the courtyard from me before we'd moved, was due shortly thereafter with her second child, a daughter. Surrounded by a small group of powerful, loving women, Andrea and her still-gestating daughter were touched by healing hands and given tokens of energy and affection in the form of beads for a bracelet Andrea could use as a focus during labor.

Midway through the evening, we gathered in the kitchen of the host, Andrea's friend Jennifer, for food and drink. She bustled around in front of the stove and returned with a steaming ceramic bowl of refried black beans smelling strongly of garlic. We all slathered crunchy, oversized tortilla chips called *tostadas* with the savory beans, and I knew that—perhaps in no small part due to the circumstances heavy with community and women's energy—I'd fallen in love with a food. It was salty and crunchy, savory with an earthy flavor that melded beautifully with the oil Jennifer had drizzled into the pot. On the table in the center of the kitchen were bowls of sliced raw onion, chunks of avocado, and shredded cheese, but I happily ate mine with just beans and tostada, helping after helping, the simple meal filling me in the warm kitchen.

After Sammi's diagnosis with EoE all those years later, I was standing tearfully in front of a stack of tortillas in the grocery store and reading "shared equipment" warnings that disqualified even the corn tortillas. Despondent, I looked up to see tostadas on the top shelf. I remembered the heady lushness and intensity in the room during the blessingway ceremony, crowded with women brushing Andrea's hair, massaging lotion into her hands, singing and chanting to welcome her baby, and then emerging into the kitchen where silky beans and spicy garlic filled a hunger I hadn't even realized I was feeling. Remembering it all, I reached up to look at the bag of crunchy tostadas. *Contains: corn, salt, lime.* All acceptable, with no warnings of shared equipment with any of our forbidden foods.

Corn tostadas and refried black beans became a go-to dish for my family that year and they have remained a staple ever since. There is no meal as simple and satisfying. We have nearly endless variations to top the beans: sliced avocado; a variety of salsas; chopped mango, corn, and tomatoes; olives; cucumber; and whatever cheeses were allowed by the medically restrictive diets we've followed.

During the year of the six-food elimination diet for eosinophilic esophagitis, it was one of the few meals I could make that could be ready in fewer than thirty minutes. A stack of tostadas fit neatly in a reusable plastic container, and so did a family-sized portion of refried beans. All the accoutrements could be carried along, too. The entire meal is even tasty at room temperature, so we dragged it to every public event where food would be served.

Most importantly for us, this meal does not seem strange to most people. It's easy for each person at our table to customize a serving to their liking, and having this in our family repertoire allowed us to avoid what might have been the worst part of any of these intensely restrictive diets we've had to follow: isolation. When Andrea's friend showed me how to press fresh garlic cloves into a can of store-bought refried black beans, how to drizzle it with oil and mix it in a pot on the stove, she did so in a kitchen filled with other people steeped in joy and support. She anointed this meal a community affair, and so it remained. No one we love and know well has gone without eating this meal with us, and to my knowledge, no one has regretted trying it.

This meal was blessed from the start with the union of loving spirits, not unlike all my other early favorite foods to prepare: my grandmother's kugel, my mother's matzo ball soup, Hilary's challah. When I cooked tostadas during the strange heartache of the year of elimination diets, I never really cooked alone.

5

EGG, SOY, NUTS, WHEAT, MILK, AND JOY, ALL MISSING

During the first phase of this elimination diet that would take the better part of a year, I was just starting to get a handle on how to feed us when Sammi's fifth birthday arrived. Sammi was accustomed to spending all her and Ronni's birthdays with David's entire family: her grandmother, aunt and uncle, great-aunts and -uncles, and cousins. It was one thing to cook without dairy, eggs, soy, nuts, and wheat for Sammi; it was quite another to do it for a whole party, which is the task that suddenly faced me.

Regardless of the challenge ahead, I was unwavering on the topic of a birthday cake. I emailed a friend from high school who owned a bakery and asked how she would approach a customer who had the food restrictions Sammi was managing. "How would you make a cake without dairy, eggs, soy, nuts, or wheat?" I asked.

She wrote back quickly, "I wouldn't. That's too hard."

If a professional baker wasn't up for the job, reason would dictate that I shouldn't feel guilty for giving up, too, but I was far from reasonable. Looking ahead at a period of restriction that would encompass Sammi's entire first year of elementary school, I refused to let her birthday pass without a cake. I scoured the internet again, googling "birthday cake eosinophilic esophagitis" and "birthday cake six food elimination diet." The results were disheartening. They featured cardboard boxes full of Smarties sugar candies beautifully wrapped so they would look like cakes; painted Styrofoam blocks with hundreds of Dum-Dums lollipops stuck into them; or mountains of shaved ice colored with Day-Glo sugar syrups and topped with tall candles.

These cakes represented children not allowed to eat anything but salt and sugar and specialty prescription liquid formulas, those who had failed all the phases of the elimination diet because every single food they tried resulted in patches of eosinophils. I ached for those children and their parents, but we were not among them, at least not yet. I refused to give in and make a cake out of anything that was not real food. It was during this time that our friend Christine surprised us by making crispy rice treats to share with Sammi at camp, using gluten-free rice cereal, soy-free margarine, and regular marshmallows (which miraculously were safe during all phases of the diet). It gave me an idea: could I add frosting to crispy rice treats? Could I decorate them?

Brief online research turned up several cakes made with crisp rice cereal, and my heart soared. I *could* make Sammi a birthday cake!

The morning of our family party, I put together the best allergen-free celebration I could. Scheduled for midafternoon so that no one would expect a meal, I started with the crisp rice "cake." There were two brands of crisp rice cereal that met our needs, and one of them was cocoa flavored. I made two batches of "treats," pressed into the pan in alternating flavors, then chilled. For the frosting, I used shortening and soy-free margarine mixed with powdered sugar and vanilla extract.

I asked my sister-in-law, Sammi's Aunt Sherri, to come early and help me decorate it. Sherri had been taking cake decorating classes and knew all kinds of techniques I didn't. The two of us pored over photos of Sammi's favorite TV show at the time, *Yo Gabba Gabba!* Carefully, we colored several bowls of the frosting in different colors to represent the backdrop from TV and then added plastic figurines from the show on top.

I stepped back and studied our work. It looked as pretty as any store-bought cake, at least before we sliced it. I breathed a sigh of relief. In the years to come, when Sammi's diet became unrestricted, I would make towering layer cakes with custard fillings, crushed Oreo cookies, fresh fruit, lemon curd, or chocolate ganache, hovering over them with my favorite decorator, Ronni. But during that wretched year of the elimination diet, crisp rice treats with frosting seemed like the height of creativity in pastry, my first-ever homemade birthday cake.

Next, I made fruit punch in a big glass pitcher with raspberries and strawberries floating in it and popped a huge bowl of popcorn, which I covered in my own homemade caramel—more soy-free margarine and lots of brown sugar, plus more vanilla.

Finally, I chopped a mountain of melon, strawberries, and mango into a big bowl. While I chopped, Sammi sat at the counter picking at her lunch and singing to our birthday gift to her—a little aquarium with two aquatic frogs in it. Between songs, she begged for bites of mango.

At the party, David's family members politely nibbled at our strange and certainly overly sweet "cake" and congratulated me on somehow making Sammi's birthday look mostly normal.

Though Sammi had been charmed by the cake and happy to have her family there, I spent the whole time anxious about whether she would, at some point, be sad about the lack of "real" cake or any of the other foods we'd normally share at a family gathering. I watched her carefully for signs of disappointment, desperate to keep anything from making her sad on her birthday. Thankfully, nothing did. The party ended before dinner, family members filing out as I tried to take a breath of relief.

But my agitation never really ended. Before school began that fall, I had met with her principal to create a 504 plan—a legal document for students with medical concerns—in which I was adamant that no one feed her anything I didn't send from home. Unfortunately, on two occasions, I found out she'd been offered unsafe treats by adults who should have known better. I was so angry that I could barely form coherent thoughts; just one mistake during any phase of this diet meant starting that six-week phase over again, since the results could be contaminated by just one bite of something forbidden—even by a "safe food" that had been made on equipment shared with something forbidden. Thankfully, Sammi had remembered my rule better than her school principal, who offered her a popsicle, or her gym teacher, who offered her a cookie, and she'd refused to take either. I held her tight and apologized for their missteps, promised her a safe version of each forbidden item, and wrote scathing emails to the district health clerks.

For her part, though, Sammi was unaffected by my churning worry. After all, she still had fruit and refried black beans, two of her favorite things. She missed her macaroni and cheese, but even that didn't seem to affect her much. She woke up every morning before kindergarten that fall, watched as I poured rice milk on her Fruity Pebbles (another miraculously "safe" find), ate half a tiny bowl, and went to school, seemingly unaffected by all of the things to which she'd have to say "no" all day.

The truth was that her life around food was largely unchanged, at least on a macro level. She arrived at her little seat in the kitchen every morning and the dinner table every night and had a bowl or plate of food set in front of her—all without having to think or act in any way. For me, though, the world had shrunk to contain nothing but food, day and night. I woke in the morning and immediately began planning the day around meal preparation. I lay in bed, hearing my daughters getting dressed and making their way downstairs, and was instantly plunged into a mental scan of my cabinets. Breakfast was the easiest—cold cereal or hot oat bran, which we'd learned was higher in protein than cream of rice. The lunch she took to school was almost always the same, too—a corn tortilla (made on uncontaminated equipment) with refried black beans and shredded vegan cheese; some raspberries in a little plastic container; a baggie of allergen-free potato chips; and a reusable juice box of rice milk mixed with chocolate syrup. During the school week, I really only needed to worry about dinner.

Most people who are in charge of making dinner for their families probably do some version of my daily meal rumination, too, thinking through what they have and how they'll put it together, whether they need to stop at the store on the way home from work for a missing ingredient or a crusty bread to go with the stew. Even those people, though, likely begin thinking about dinner many hours later than I did that year. From the moment I awoke until I put the last clean, dry dish back in the cupboard before bed, I thought about cooking. Had I double-checked to be sure the spice blend I'd bought for the lentils wasn't made on shared equipment with any of our "forbidden" ingredients? Did the chickpea flour for the crepes need to be at room temperature before I used it? Did I have enough onions? If I had only two pots that had been sterilized at the start of the diet, and I needed three to make the soup, the rice, and the pudding, should I make the rice in the afternoon and store it in one of my sterilized plastic containers so that I could make the pudding during dinner? If I was going to do that, I'd need to be home by 12:30, and if I dropped the kids off for school at 9:00, then I'd really only get three hours of work at the coffeeshop, where my scone—my beloved, crucial scone—was waiting.

And all that was *after* I'd already brought home the ingredients. Grocery shopping was an hours-long ordeal now, since I had to read ingredients so carefully. Although doctors who treat children with eosinophilic esophagitis have differing opinions on the strictness required, Sammi's doctor insisted that she not only avoid the listed foods, but also avoid any foods made on shared equipment with those foods. I had to read every label carefully, standing in every aisle of the store squinting and running my finger down the ingredient lists. One night around 3:00 a.m., I sat up in bed and said aloud, "no, it has soy protein isolate." David stirred next to me, and I realized where I was. My heart pounding, I tried fruitlessly to fall back to sleep.

I took Sammi to the store with me only once during the first phase of the diet. It was her last week at preschool because she'd soon be starting the summer day camp near our new house to meet other incoming kindergarteners. She wanted to bring a "last day" treat, but without cupcakes or ice cream allowed on the diet, our options were very limited. She had decided on candy. I cleared it with the teacher, who was already feeding Sammi only from little plastic containers I gave her every morning. I thought it must be strange for Sammi to watch her friends eating graham crackers and juice boxes while she ate the little tub of berries I'd sent, but she wasn't complaining. This candy treat seemed like a very reasonable reward for her patience.

In the candy aisle, I crouched in front of her, holding a bag of Smarties in one hand and a bag of Dum-Dums lollipops in the other. After all my research, it seemed these were the only candies that were allowed during the six-food elimination diet. Sammi carefully considered which one to choose, squinting and tapping her finger on her chin, a funny little gesture she'd started using at the age of two.

"I don't know which one to pick," she said, finally. "You can pick, Momma."

I looked at the packages and felt a wave of deep sadness come over me. Sammi was being so reasonable, not even begging for the chocolates or the gummy bears or any of the other fun candies around us. I'd told her what was possible, and she'd simply accepted it. Blinking away tears, I tucked both bags under one arm and squeezed her into my side with the other.

"You know what?" I asked her. "Let's get both."

She broke into a big smile and clapped her hands. "Really?" she squealed.

"Yes, really. Just this once," I promised and got to my feet.

Standing just a few feet away from us, an older woman furrowed her eyebrows at me as we got nearer. "Excuse me," she said. "But I have to tell you: all that sugar isn't good for a little girl."

Just as quickly as the wave of sadness had rushed over me, a new wave of burning rage crested now.

"Well," I hissed. "She can't have dairy, eggs, soy, nuts, or wheat. You want to take away sugar, too?"

The woman's eyes widened, and she clucked her tongue. "Oh my goodness. I had no idea."

I scowled. "Well, then maybe you shouldn't judge strangers in the grocery store, huh?" I pulled Sammi closer to me and said, loud enough for the woman to hear, "Kiddo, that's what we call a rude busybody. This candy is fine for you to share with your friends."

I was angry for days after that, but Sammi, as usual, just let it go.

Given the stringency of this diet, I would have thought I'd have more support from the dietician we'd met in the gastroenterologist's office, but she was barely any use. She'd mailed us a huge packet of information after Sammi was diagnosed, but during our first meeting, it was clear to me that my own research already had outpaced her knowledge.

"It looks like a lot of the foods on this list are meat," I said, "but the doctor told us not to add meat to Sammi's diet because she's never had it before."

"That's right," she agreed, "we don't want to complicate the potential results of her tests by adding a new food."

"That's what I *just said*," I responded, frustrated already. "But this packet you sent with all the suggested foods is mostly meat. So what do you recommend for us?"

"Well, that's the packet we send to all new patients. Obviously, your situation is different. You'll want to also avoid the foods in there that have meat in them."

I turned to David, who was holding Sammi on his lap, and widened my eyes. He looked over the top of Sammi's fluffy blond hair and said, "So, what you're saying is that we're kind of on our own as far as figuring out what to feed her? Just follow this list but without the meat?"

"No, no," the dietician assured us. "I'm here for you! Any questions you have, I'm always happy to answer. What do you want to know?"

I wanted to say: *How to feed her. What to feed her. Why she still pockets bites of food and sips of water in her cheeks like a chipmunk. Why her symptoms aren't anything like the list of symptoms of other kids with EoE. How to make her grow. How to get through six weeks on this joy-free diet.*

Instead, I said, "Any recommendations for denser foods she can eat?"

The dietician rifled through the pages of the packet—already worn and dog-eared from my own frantic looking—and said, "Have you ever tried beans?"

The conversation ended soon thereafter. I went home to my own cookbooks and spent hours cross-legged on the floor, marking pages with sticky notes labeled "sub coconut milk for cream" and "sub flax meal + water for eggs" and "OK without the peanut sauce." Inspired by an acquaintance whose daughter was newly diagnosed with celiac disease, I filled a notebook with the names and page numbers of recipes I wanted to try from each of my vegan cookbooks and then made a chart with each of our names. We rated each recipe on a scale of "bleccchh!" to "definitely make again." I began my meal planning on Sundays, including notes about how to make the ingredients that would go into the recipes I was trying: blends of different kinds of gluten-free flours; soaked seeds and dried beans; items thickened with agar that needed time in the fridge.

"How do people do this?" I sniffled one day to my friend Andrea. "There has to be someone out there who has figured this out better than I have."

She put her hand on my knee and said, "I don't think most people would do this the way you're doing it, though."

I asked her what she meant, and she explained. "I just think, if this was me, I'd find three or four things that Sammi could eat, and I'd make just those things for the next six weeks, and the rest of us would eat normally. I wouldn't be as creative as you're trying to be. I'd just . . . make it simple."

The truth was that I would have loved to do that, but something stopped me from turning food into nothing more than fuel. Sure, I could have given Sammi gluten-free noodles and tomato sauce; lentil soup; and corn tortillas with refried beans for six weeks, and she might not have minded, but something had changed in me when it came to cooking. All those summer months at the farmers market—not to mention our subscription to a local CSA that gave us a box of vegetables directly from a farm twenty weeks of the year—had turned food into something more sacred. It was creative for me, after all this time, exciting and steeped in history and pride. When I first mixed a homemade vegan/gluten-free cheese sauce with a box of gluten-free noodles, topped it with homemade paprika-seasoned gluten-free breadcrumbs, and then baked it in a pan, I hadn't just followed a recipe: I'd resurrected macaroni and cheese for my daughter in a format she could eat. I had slayed a mighty beast. I had *won*.

Aside from that, I'd spent much of my childhood uneasy as my parents watched my brother and me eat the foods they couldn't. When my father was on a mostly liquid weight-loss diet program during one of our long summer road trips, I remember sitting at roadside diners eating grilled cheese sandwiches while he sipped a cup of black coffee. Back in the car, he ate piece after piece of sugar-free hard candy. I'd dig through the bag we stowed between our seats to find him a coffee-flavored one, and the smell in the car was a mix of the sourness of ketosis, coffee, and artificial sweetener. I'd feel guilty about my sandwich and snacks as I watched my father sip his coffee, drink his diet shakes, and eat his one salad every evening.

My mother, too, was always on a diet, usually Weight Watchers. "I just want to *smell* your chocolate," she'd say to me as I ate Hershey's Special Dark from my bag of Halloween candy in middle school. I watched her watching my brother and me line up chocolate chips on the raised edge of our dining room table, occasionally asking for "just one" from each of us. I knew that she wanted more but she wasn't allowed; for her, the "nothing tastes as good as being thin feels" sign on the fridge was gospel. As a child, I didn't know that the person who wouldn't allow her to eat the chocolate or my father to have lunch was not some distant authority figure—they were on their own continual self-imposed path toward weight loss—so I felt oddly unworthy and wrong for eating "normal" food while they watched, obviously wanting it, too.

Because of that, when Sammi was put on the six-food elimination diet, I found I could not bring myself to sit at the table and eat the things she was not allowed, even if so many of her favorites were still safe for her. I couldn't bear the guilt of it. Sammi was easygoing so, in retrospect, I'm convinced she would have been fine with us snacking on "forbidden" items when she was nearby, but I was resolute: we were in this together. We would eat together as a family. End of story. We snuck Ronni over to friends' houses for pizza and cookies; David ate lunch out every workday; and I had my morning scone and mocha. And so, through the full elimination diet and all the phases that followed: adding eggs, then soy, then nuts, then wheat, and finally dairy, we progressed as a team.

We weren't alone, though. Help came from every corner of our little world, from my mother-in-law and sister-in-law, who scoured their local health food stores for safe foods for Sammi and cooked things she could eat in freshly sterilized pots and pans; to my friends Amy and Ben whose daughter was in kindergarten with Sammi and who made sure that they provided Sammi-safe snacks for the whole class when it was their turn; to Christine who not only made crispy rice treats but also huge pots of lentils and rice so we could all have dinner together. When my parents found out that Jelly Belly jelly beans were allergen free, they sent Sammi a tub so big that they lasted all year.

On the days of the endoscopies, which marked the end of each phase of the diet, my friend Clare, whose daughter was Ronni's best friend, received Ronni at five in the morning, wrapping her in her arms and ushering her inside to eat breakfast with them and walk with them to school so that David and I could take Sammi to the hospital together. At the hospital, David's mother Susan was always waiting for us, ready to entertain Sammi as we completed paperwork. She stayed with us while we waited for each procedure to be finished and then left when we met Sammi in recovery each time, giving Sammi a kiss goodbye and then leaving us to wait together as Sammi rose back to the surface of consciousness, sleepy and often with a sore throat.

Those endoscopy days were hard, and their early morning scheduling often meant that David went back to work as soon as Sammi was released. He'd make sure we made it to the car and then took a cab to his office. I'd drive home with Sammi in the back seat, listening to her favorite Junie B. Jones book recordings, tears streaming down my face.

Being the only one to go into the operating room with her—to stay with her until she was fully unconscious—felt like the right thing to do, but I never became numb to the experience. In the room, of course, I'd be cheery and dry-eyed. I'd hold Sammi's hand as we wheeled down the hallway to the operating room, wearing my surgical "bunny suit" and hat, chatting about what movie we might watch later when we got home. I'd watch as the nurses settled her on the gurney and double-checked that they'd smeared the inside of the rubber mask with the strawberry-scented oil so that, when the bitter sevoflurane anesthesia gas mixed with the oxygen, it would be disguised by the smell of berries. Then I'd put my hand on hers and sing to her: sometimes the same lullabies I sang every night at bedtime, sometimes pop songs she was learning in her ukulele lessons, sometimes my own favorites that I'd sung when she was a baby. As she stared into my eyes and anesthetic gas began to fill her mask, sometimes she'd fight to keep her eyes open. Other times, her eyes would roll up into her head, her mouth would froth, and she'd try fruitlessly to reach up and pull off the mask, her body going limp and ineffectual from the anesthesia. The whole time, I kept singing and looking her in the eye, calm and without a waver in my voice. When the anesthesiologist confirmed she was totally asleep, I'd kiss Sammi's cheek and walk out of the room.

Though this was the easiest way to give a child anesthesia—the IV needle with general anesthesia wasn't even inserted until the gas had knocked her out—it was also almost impossible, as a Jewish woman, to watch my daughter be put to sleep with gas and not think about the Holocaust. And each time I walked out of the room, knowing I was going down the hallway to David and Susan who had lost, respectively, a father and husband in surgery, I knew I had to arrive in that room with my emotions in check. So during those walks from the operating room to the waiting room, I sucked all my emotions back in. It was not until the drive home, alone in the front seat where not even Sammi could see my face, that I could let go. We'd spend the afternoon on the couch together, snuggling and watching movies. I would often wrap my hand around her ankle and fall asleep with my head pressed into her hip, exhausted but vigilant to her every movement.

But all that would have been worth it if not for the gnawing, not-quite-right feeling I had as Sammi "passed" food trial after food trial, an indication that the foods we were adding were not the ones causing damage to her esophagus. After she passed the egg and soy trials—giving us an amazing number of new options for dinner every night—we thought for certain nuts would prove to be the culprit. She hated them—even peanut butter—and always had. "Maybe her body knows these are the bad guys," I'd told David as we counted out the minimum number of tree nuts and peanuts she needed to eat each day of the trial. It was a daily struggle as she squeezed her eyes shut and dutifully chewed each cashew, chasing every nut with a gulp of water she pouched in her cheeks.

But she passed the nut trial, too. At our clinic appointment before beginning the wheat trial, I asked her doctor whether her surprising lack of typical EoE symptoms surprised him.

"She never vomits," I said as Sammi sat on the exam table wearing big headphones and watching a movie on a portable DVD player. "She's only ever thrown up once in her life, when she was choking on an edamame pod." Children with EoE were notorious for vomiting regularly.

"It's unusual," he admitted, "but not unheard of."

"And she's still not even really underweight," I pressed him. That was true, too. She was tiny—barely clinging to the bottom 2 percent of the growth chart—but she was proportionate. Her 2 percent in weight mirrored her 2 percent in height, and even through the most restrictive phase of this diet, she had not lost any ground. It was a full-time job to keep her fed, but I had so far proved that I was up for it. Regardless of all that, I listened to the nurses cluck their tongues when we weighed Sammi at the beginning of each appointment.

"Still 'failure to thrive,'" they'd say as Sammi hopped off the scale, setting off my now-routine "failure to feed" inner monologue. I'd vow to myself that at the next appointment, Sammi would have gained a little more weight, grown a little taller. I'd redouble my efforts to find foods she liked that would nourish her into a child who managed to "thrive."

Back with the gastroenterologist, he answered, "Well, you're right that she's not skinny. But she is pretty small, isn't she?"

I nodded. "Is there any chance," I asked, not for the first time, "that this has something to do with her double aortic arch from when she was a baby?"

The doctor kept tapping away at his electronic notes. "This disease only really correlates with gastro-esophageal reflux, and even that, we don't know which comes first. A chicken-egg thing, you know?"

And so we proceeded into the wheat trial—a glorious binge of baked goods and regular pasta—shocked to find eventually that she passed that one, too. Dairy had to be the culprit, and I was more than a little relieved. I'd been baking and cooking without dairy for myself for years. This I could do!

But even better than giving me the opportunity to make my own baked goods, the wheat trial had offered something extraordinary. For the first time in ten months, I could also buy store-bought baked goods for Sammi. The first week of the wheat trial, I picked up both girls from school in my car and told them that we were going on a surprise adventure.

"Did you bring us a snack?" Ronni asked me.

"No," I said. "Just wait."

The drive to the nearest kosher bakery—where all baked goods are made *parve,* a Hebrew word that indicated they were made completely without dairy—was less than ten minutes, during which time Ronni and Sammi tried to guess where we were going. As they chattered, my thoughts were consumed by the ready-to-eat pastries awaiting us.

"Are we getting new Webkinz?" they asked, eyes wide as they pictured the little stuffed animals that came with online codes to activate their animated counterparts.

"You have enough Webkinz," I answered over my shoulder.

"Are we visiting Tian and Amanda?" Ronni suggested, recognizing the street where we often turned to visit my friend Andrea's children.

"No, not that," I replied.

They went on and on, whispering, guessing, giggling and shedding mittens and hats between them in the back seat. When I pulled over on the side of the road across from the bakery, they both looked around, confused.

"Where are we?" they both asked.

"Look across the street," I said, a huge grin forming on my face.

Sammi looked across the street, back at me, across the street again. "I don't know," she said.

Ronni couldn't figure out what we were looking at, either. I took them by the hand, one on each side of me, and raced us through a break in the traffic to the door of the bakery. When I opened it and ushered them inside, they still didn't look as though they understood what was happening. I knelt in front of them.

"You know how we added wheat back in to Sammi's diet?" I asked. They both nodded and I continued. "The only thing Sammi can't have now is dairy, and this bakery doesn't make anything with dairy. Everything here is safe for Sammi. Everything."

Ronni's eyes widened and a smile broke across her face. "Wow!"

"So," I went on, "You guys can pick out any treat you want for right now, and something else to bring to school in your lunch tomorrow. Go look!"

Ronni took Sammi by the hand and said, "Come on, Sammi! Let's pick two things we both like and share!"

Sammi didn't say anything and looked no more excited than before she knew why we were here. She dutifully picked out rainbow sprinkle cookies and chocolate cupcakes to share with Ronni, but I could see that this was not nearly as thrilling for her as it was for Ronni or even for me. She nibbled at the cookie in the car, no happier than she was with any other food I'd given her that day.

"Is it good, Sunshine?" I asked from the front seat.

"Mmm-hmm," she answered. "It's really good."

There was a pause, and then she asked, "Was that the surprise, Mommy?"

The truth of it was that the treat was really for me. It was about not having to bake the items myself and about the beauty of leaving the house for a treat if we wanted one. For Sammi, delicious food appeared on her plate as often as I could make it. I rationalized her lack of real enthusiasm with the fact that, at age five, it really doesn't matter whether the food comes from a restaurant or Mommy's kitchen.

Ronni, on the other hand, had some sense at age eight that all this cooking was time consuming and challenging for me. I seldom had as much time as before to play Candyland, color, or read with her and Sammi. I was always going to the grocery store on the weekends, poring over cookbooks and websites, and saying "I need a few more minutes to watch this on the stove" when anyone asked me questions between the hours of three and six. Ronni had some sense of the magnitude of a bakery visit and, besides, had a much more active sweet tooth.

I knew just how much she appreciated our visit to the bakery at bedtime. She and I lay together in her bed for me to hear her three "happy thoughts"—a gratitude ritual we'd started when she was very small. For her last happy thought, she mentioned the bakery.

"My third happy thought," she announced through a yawn, "is going to the bakery with you and Sammi."

"Was that cupcake yummy?" I asked.

"It was good," she said, "but it's also a happy thought because you didn't have to make a snack today."

"Why is that happy?" I asked. "Don't I make yummy snacks?" I fake growled, tickling her armpits.

"Yes! You make yummy snacks!" she said, laughing. "But today you only had to make dinner, and so we got to go to the bakery right after school and sing songs in the car."

I leaned over and nuzzled the top of her head, smelling her shampoo and feeling the thick waves against my cheek. Ronni, I realized, was paying more attention than it seemed.

"I cook a lot, huh?" I said into her hair.

She nodded.

"I know this is hard," I said, curling my body around hers. "I know making all this food that's safe for Sammi is really, really hard, and you have to eat a lot of weird stuff you don't always like."

"It's OK, Mommy," she said.

"Yeah, it's OK, but it's a lot of work for me and for you. You are a wonderful, wonderful big sister, and a super-awesome daughter. Do you know that?"

"Yeah," she answered.

"I hope so," I murmured in the dark. "Because it's totally true."

Sammi went on to pass her wheat trial a month later, moving on to the dairy one. Before the final endoscopy, which we knew would end in a relapse of her EoE, we fed Sammi on ice cream, cream cheese, and pot after pot of her favorite neon orange boxed macaroni and cheese. The fresh bloom of eczema across her arms and legs made me even more certain that dairy was the offender, and when we went in for her last endoscopy, the doctor nodded.

"Sure looks like her body doesn't like all this dairy," he said.

For the seventh time in twelve months, I walked her back into the operating room, grateful that we'd soon know for sure what was wrong, begin avoiding dairy again, and move on with our lives. When, just ninety minutes later in the recovery room, the doctor showed us photos he'd taken of her smooth, pink, unblemished esophagus, we didn't know what to think.

"It looks OK," I said, incredulous. "Doctor, what do you think?"

He smiled at me and slid the photos back into his folder. "I agree with you."

"So . . . what does this mean?" David asked.

The doctor shrugged. "I think it means she passed this trial, too. We have to wait for the biopsies, but, you know, it looks good."

We were dumbstruck as he shook our hands and walked away. Before he pushed open the door of the recovery suite, I stopped him.

"Wait, doctor," I called. "What do we feed her now?"

He winked at me from the doorway. "Everything," he said.

6

CHINESE FOOD, IN A HURRY

O n June 22, 2011, I sent this email message to more than fifty of our friends and family members.

Subject: We always thought Sammi was a miracle . . .

. . . and now she has gone and proved it to us.

Today, the gastroenterologist told us that Sammi is now the third child he's ever seen whose eosinophilic esophagitis has gone into total remission. Her diet is completely as it was before this all began, and her esophagus is healthy. He called it "wonderful and rare." I think I'm going to go ahead and call it a miracle.

This is not the end of the road—though one of the other children in the practice has remained in this type of remission for almost five years now, there is still not enough research on this disease to be able to prove that it can be "cured." He referred to it as "remission" and wants to see Sammi in six months and to do another endoscopy in a year. Assuming she doesn't become ill, she'll probably just be scoped once a year. We need to now try to get her off of her proton pump inhibitor (reflux medication). But we can do that while she enjoys an unrestricted diet, and that is a gift. We can stop putting her under general anesthesia every six weeks, and that is an incredible gift. We are amazingly, amazingly grateful. . . .

With love,

Debi, David, Ronni, and Sammi

My mother-in-law Susan said, "Didn't I tell you she was going to be one of the rare ones who healed completely?"

The congratulations poured in. People thanked G-d, praised our courage under pressure, extolled Sammi's bravery and good nature, and suggested gluttonous celebrations. We felt celebrated by our community; everyone was relieved that Sammi was healed.

Privately—and despite my cheery email message—I wasn't buying it. I began to do my own research. In all the groups I'd joined and the studies I'd read online, I found no evidence that eosinophilic esophagitis could be spontaneously cured. There were no other children like Sammi out there, or at least none whose parents were sharing their stories on the internet or whose doctors had written about it in medical journals. I posted our story in one online forum and was met with tepid congratulations from some parents—likely written as they worried over their own children—and nothing from anyone else whose story was similar. I lurked in those groups for a while, and then, as the months went on, slowly unsubscribed.

The truth was that I assumed Sammi would relapse, and I didn't want to live in the future those forums revealed. All the data predicted it; evidence abounded in all the stories of parents waxing nostalgic for the years when their children could eat ten or twelve different foods and now were limited to just elemental formula. I had virtually no hope that our life would remain as easy as it was now. I moved through the months of June and July in what was likely a fog of postcrisis weariness. People who knew what we'd experienced greeted me with hoots of joy and questions about all the food Sammi must be eating now, but I found myself unable to shake my sense of impending doom.

I needed something to get my mojo back. I'd spent a year cooking for survival; on a whim, I bought a totally frivolous series of dessert cookbooks and began cooking for fun. I bought piping tools and decorated cupcakes with colored flowers and swirls. I made "cowgirl cookies" with nuts and coconut and chocolate; cinnamony snickerdoodles; lemon sugar cookies with glittery yellow sprinkles; and rocky road cookies with dairy-free white chocolate chips I found at a kosher grocery store. My own lactose intolerance was now our only restriction. I learned to cook dried figs into a paste to make homemade fig bars. I made peanut butter blondies and dark chocolate brownies, rich pie-pan shortbread and light-as-a-feather chocolate pillows filled with fluffy peanut butter filling.

I baked my way through August and September. Once I'd made my way through every interesting recipe in my cookie and cupcake cookbooks and pushed the unused bags of strange ingredients to the back of the cupboard, I felt like I had a normal kitchen again. I had baked my way from defiance into joy.

By the time Sammi started first grade, we were settled into normal life with a normal kid. Despite the fact that we'd made it through a year of highly unusual food and regular hospital visits, Sammi seemed like every other kid in her class aside from being a full head shorter and looking at least a year younger. She was spunky and fun, with a squeaky high voice and a pixie cut of honey-colored hair. She took ukulele lessons and played soccer. Her teachers complained that she was often too chatty, but I appreciated her social nature. I felt myself relax.

During that first grade year, I began—for the first time since Sammi was born—to ponder what I wanted to do with my own time. I'd planned to do this soul-searching a year prior but instead had spent every spare minute of Sammi's kindergarten year in the pursuit or preparation of safe food. Now I looked at the minimal web design work I was doing and made efforts to grow my freelance business. I attended a technology conference for the first time since leaving my job when she was a baby. I bought a new laptop, freshened up stagnating skills, and started to shake the dust off my professional mind.

During the previous grueling year—in fact, the previous grueling *six* years—all my energy had been concentrated on keeping my family functioning, and a good chunk of my mind always was skimming through my mental notes about Sammi's health. Though all parents are changed irreversibly when their children arrive, my world had been upended in every way. My plans for my own future had veered off course, and—even if I'd wanted to—I couldn't return to my previous job now that our lives were built around my flexible freelance work. Whomever I would be now, aside from David's wife and Ronni and Sammi's mother, it would be a vastly different version of myself than I'd planned before Sammi was born.

Midway through this year—Sammi in first and Ronni in fourth grade—I began to run outside in the early mornings before the girls woke for school, reclaiming moments I'd previously used to plan meals. The moment I reached the shore of Lake Michigan was always magnificent: both peaceful and, on closer inspection, alive with the churning, rolling waves and raucous seagulls. Like the lake, I seemed calm and steady, but there were depths of fear and crests of panic that I'd stifled. I stood on the beach some days, panting, watching the surface endlessly changing.

One day, I stood on the beach and stared at the horizon. There were limits, regardless of my perseverance; I could go no further east than the water. It was best to accept this and turn in a different direction. Having been offered no real contextual discussion with anyone on Sammi's medical team, I instinctively planned my life around the need for flexibility and vigilance. With nowhere to put that watchful energy, I ran, looping my neighborhood from the Chicago River to Lake Michigan, thinking about what had happened and what was going to happen next. Despite the doctors' optimism, those meditative miles could not take me far from my intuition. I was anxious to my core. *Something is still wrong*, I thought, pushing it down into my feet.

On the surface, though, everything looked relatively calm for most of Sammi's first grade year. It wasn't until late spring—nearly a year after her last endoscopy—when I began to notice Sammi's mealtime behavior was getting worse.

The four of us had always eaten dinner together around our dining room table, chatting and sharing stories, laughing and joking. Every night, after twenty minutes or so, Ronni, David, and I would be finished, but Sammi was always still eating, slowly, often poised in midsentence with food on her fork, gesturing with the bite of broccoli that she had been holding for many minutes.

Unlike families I knew who struggled with a picky child at mealtimes, Sammi's issues were seldom the refusal to eat what was on her plate. In fact, if we suggested that she might be finished, she'd often tell us that she wasn't. She'd take a bite, chew it slowly, and begin a conversation. Five or six minutes later, we'd realize she wasn't using the moments when someone else was talking to take another bite—instead, she was watching, nodding, interacting, but not eating any more.

"Pick up your fork and put some food on it," David or I would say, rolling our eyes.

An hour after sitting down, Sammi still would be spearing pieces of food, now cold. By then, Ronni would be playing or reading a book in a chair nearby. David or I would have escaped to the kitchen to do dishes. The parent left at the table might start reading to Sammi or to him- or herself in an effort to stave off the frustration of still sitting there.

By the fall of Sammi's second grade year, this scene would still be unfolding after ninety minutes. We'd begin a countdown to the end of the meal, dinnertime edging right into bedtime. We never had time to play board games, watch a television show, or take a walk after dinner. We seldom had "picnic" dinners in front of a movie, lest we adults lose our focus or vigilance over the state of Sammi's plate. Dinner would begin with my excitement over the meal I'd made—often tailored to provide dense nutrition in every bite, to appeal to Ronni's slowly narrowing palate, and to avoid dairy for my lactose intolerance—and end with me at the very edge of my patience, nagging Sammi in a tone barely masking my growing aggravation.

In addition, Sammi was increasingly returning to a familiar practice that had been giving us pause for years. She would stop eating a few bites into a meal to go to the kitchen, get a cup, and fill it with water. When she returned to the table, she took gulps of water with which she filled her cheeks like a chipmunk. A little at a time, she swallowed the water in tiny portions. Sometimes, she'd return to refill her cup several times during a meal.

It seemed wrong. I sat there, night after night, staring at Sammi eating in slow motion, musing and, despite myself, fuming, and it was even worse when school began. If the problem of dinnertime butting against bedtime was irritating, the problem of breakfast time butting into the morning school bell was excruciating. We could delay bedtime if we wanted, but that bell was nonnegotiable.

Every morning, I gave Sammi a bowl of her favorite cereal and reminded her that we needed to leave for school in one hour. As she and Ronni chatted over their breakfast, I began making Sammi's lunch. I tried hard to make every bite as calorie dense as I could, since, despite her remission, she was not growing any more quickly, leaving "failure to thrive" still at the top of her medical chart. Sometimes I put a chopped and salted avocado in a plastic container atop an ice pack. Other times, I gave her a solid piece of milk chocolate. The most important thing I gave her, though, was that same refillable eight-ounce juice box with Carnation Instant Breakfast. I made it every morning and set it next to Sammi's cereal, which, after the fifteen minutes I'd spent making lunches, was still almost untouched.

"Sammi, please eat your cereal," I reminded her. "And here's your milk."

"Sorry, Mommy," she said every morning.

Inevitably, an hour after placing a small bowl of cereal in front of her, I would tell her we had to leave for school. She'd tell me again that she wasn't finished with breakfast yet, and I would grouchily remind her that it had been an *hour* since she started.

"Here," I'd say nearly every morning, handing her the cup of Instant Breakfast. "Drink this on the way to school."

And nearly every day, she'd take it with her, barely touching it as we walked.

The cup would come home from school in her lunch box, still half-full. I'd also find half of the half-quesadilla I gave her, most of the avocado or chocolate, and an empty container from the raspberries.

I was worried, which came out in frustrated scolding. If I forgot to check her lunch box when she came home, I'd quickly realize how little she'd eaten once she sat down to do her homework. She'd pull it out of her backpack and begin to do simple writing exercises, and within moments she'd be dissolving into angry tears.

"I don't know how to do it!" she'd say.

If I tried to help her, she'd scream and pound the counter or sometimes hit herself in the head, reminding me of the epic, head-banging tantrums of her toddler years. I'd tell her to breathe deeply and count to ten. While she was trying to collect herself, I'd reach for her lunch box and find it mostly full. I calculated roughly: since last night's dinner—which had ended at bedtime with a half-full plate—she'd eaten maybe 300 calories.

Sammi was hungry, and I knew it. I'd tell her I thought she was hungry and that's why she couldn't focus on her homework, but if I put her uneaten lunch in front of her, she would finally finish it in time for dinner, and the cycle would repeat itself again. By the time she went in for her check-up endoscopy just after Thanksgiving, it felt like food was the only topic of conversation between us, consisting almost completely of me asking whether, when, and how much she'd eaten.

"I'm full all the way to the top!" she'd cry, sitting at the kitchen counter, where we finally started bringing her while we washed dishes.

"OK, then I guess you're done after half a bowl of soup and two bites of bread?" I'd snap.

"No, I want more," she'd insist. "I'm just full all the way to my throat." And a tear would slide down her cheek, making me hate myself for my sharp tone.

It didn't make sense that she would be "full all the way to her throat" and also still want more. I thought she'd likely relapsed, as all of the literature on EoE had predicted she would. After her endoscopy, her gastroenterologist shook his head as I described the way she'd been eating.

"It does sound like a relapse," he said. Her esophagus had been riddled with white patches that day, and though we'd need to wait for the biopsy results, he thought they would prove to be eosinophils. "Let's get her back on her PPI," he said, referring to the medication Sammi had taken from her first year until just after her previous endoscopy.

PPI is an abbreviation for proton pump inhibitor, a medication that stops the stomach from producing most of the acid that leads to painful symptoms of gastric reflux like heartburn. Sammi's doctors told us to stop giving it to her after she'd gone into remission, and the process of discontinuing the medication, cold turkey, had been terrible. With no suggestions from anyone in the gastroenterology practice, I'd reached out to Sammi's pediatrician, who told us to hold tight through all her gagging and the accompanying burning pain, a kind of rebound effect from stopping the medication. We'd been given permission to supplement with Tums, but it was heartbreaking to hear a five-year-old cough, gag, and then ask in a hoarse voice, "Mommy, can I have Tums?" When the gastroenterologist decided to put her back on the PPI, my heart dropped again, knowing how hard it would be to discontinue it when the time came, but we did as we were told.

One thing was very different this time: the dosing. She'd been prescribed more than twice her previous dose. The gastroenterologist said that she could tolerate quite a bit more for her size and that he had a theory he wanted to test. We picked up the prescription from the pharmacy on our way home from the hospital that day, returning once again to the awkward schedule that the medication required.

The twice-per-day doses came in berry-flavored melting tablets that had to be administered thirty minutes before breakfast and dinner. That meant that Sammi's school day had to begin a minimum of ninety minutes before we walked out the door. I snuck into her room early and tried to get her to take it and then go back to sleep, but she always woke completely. Thirty minutes later, she could begin eating, a task that took right up until the moment we left. Sometimes, I kept her sitting at the counter in front of her cereal as I slid socks and shoes onto her feet, not wanting to waste a moment of time that she could spend eating.

Dinnertime was easier, assuming we were eating as a family at home but harder if we had plans with anyone else or were eating at a restaurant. When the gastroenterologist called to say that her biopsies showed a clear return to disease, he also said that he didn't want to change her diet again. He wanted to be absolutely sure that the eosinophil growth was not caused by stomach acid, so Sammi was scheduled for another endoscopy in January after six weeks on the PPI. Free to eat out in restaurants—perhaps, we thought, for the last time, if Sammi's diet might change soon—we did it often. I had to set alarms on my phone for thirty minutes before a meal so I could give Sammi her medicine, sometimes planning poorly and taking her for a walk to give the PPI a chance to work before she ate while everyone else started without us.

Something new became obvious just a few weeks into this new dosing regimen, though: Sammi was eating. Several times during the second week, I watched as her cereal bowl emptied more than ten minutes before we had to leave for school. Then she came home with her entire lunchtime half-quesadilla gone. "I ate it at lunch!" she said proudly. I held my breath as, one afternoon, she sat at the kitchen counter to do her homework and, unprompted, opened her lunch box to finish the container of cheesy crackers that remained.

But the most powerful proof of the magic in that high dose of PPI came while Sammi and I wandered through a bookstore in the early evening, waiting to meet Ronni and David for dinner. As I aimlessly thumbed through a stack of cookbooks, Sammi interrupted my reverie.

"Mommy," she asked, "are we going to a restaurant for dinner?"

"Mmm-hmm," I responded absentmindedly.

"When are we going?" she probed more insistently.

"After the bookstore," I said. "We'll hang out here until we're done looking."

"I'm done," she declared. "Can we leave? I want food. I'm *starving*."

I dropped to my knees, my winter coat in a pile at her ankles, and put my hands on her upper arms. "You're really hungry?" I asked.

She nodded. "*Really* hungry."

"OK," I said. "Let's go. Let's go get dinner right now."

As we made our way to the Chinese restaurant, my chest pounded when I realized that she had never once, in her entire life, spontaneously told me that she was hungry. When we arrived, we didn't wait for Ronni and David. I ordered her a plate of fried rice with vegetables and tofu, and she tucked in as though I hadn't spent the previous seven years begging her to eat. She didn't eat a huge portion, but what she ate went from plate to fork to mouth without any nagging at all. When David arrived, he and I spent the meal giving each other incredulous glances and squeezing each other's knees beneath the table.

This behavior continued during the weeks leading up to her next appointment in January. She began asking for snacks between meals, something she'd almost never done before. She ate dinner in an hour or less. She occasionally finished her Carnation Instant Breakfast before coming home from school. It felt like a miracle.

"It's just amazing," I said to the gastroenterologist before her endoscopy. "She's so improved on that medicine!"

He sat up a little taller and looked at Sammi, "You think so?" he asked me while winking at her.

"I do," I said.

The gastroenterologist explained to us that, in the time since Sammi's diagnosis with EoE, additional research had uncovered something curious. Researchers were calling this discovery PPIREE. It stands for "proton pump inhibitor responsive esophageal eosinophilia." It seemed that eosinophils in the esophagus were sometimes held at bay by proton-pump inhibitors like the one Sammi was taking. Why Sammi's eosinophils responded so well to it now versus when she was first diagnosed with EoE was confusing—perhaps it was the higher dose—but the doctor was intrigued enough by the improvement in her symptoms that he wanted to continue the high dose of the PPI, with no changes to her diet.

For the next three months, Sammi's eating habits were almost un-recognizable. Although the kinds of foods she liked best didn't change, her enthusiasm for them and the speed at which she could eat them increased dramatically. She expressed hunger more often. Breakfast ended before she needed to leave for school at least half of the time. She finished her Carnation Instant Breakfast most days. For the first time ever, we saw her eating foods other than berries with gusto.

In April, she had her tenth endoscopy. She was in complete remission again—and had gained as much weight in three months as she usually did in a whole year.

I thought we had finally solved the problem forever and blessed those little dissolving tablets every morning and evening. *We can do this forever,* I thought, *and it would be easy.* But just six weeks later, a new doctor on the team told us that we needed to try to lower Sammi's dose.

"These drugs aren't really intended to be used indefinitely," he told us, perched on the edge of his seat. "They can cause issues with bone density and vitamin absorption. We've got to see how low we can get this dose without making her sick again."

Cutting the dose in half was an immediate disaster. Within three days, Sammi was coughing and gagging again. Two days after that, she was again eating so slowly we had to bring her back to the kitchen counter as we did dishes. The next week, she sobbed at the dinner table.

"I'm just so tired of having to *eat!*" she cried. "I just want to stop eating. Can I just stop? *Please?*"

I hugged her tight, in tears myself. In the cabinet above the kitchen counter was exactly what she needed to feel better. I fired off a panicked message to the advanced practice nurse in the gastroenterology office, and they adjusted the dose from half of what had made her feel great to three-quarters.

Over the course of the next four months, we brought her down to the half-dose slowly, finally getting there by fall. She didn't gag and cough as much, but her appetite dwindled. The weight she'd gained while on the higher dose of the medication fell off, leaving dark circles below her eyes. By the time she started third grade in the fall, now eight years old and hovering around forty pounds, I was feeling helpless. Our days and nights returned to the same pattern of me trying to feed her and her pouching her cheeks full of cup after cup of water. Night after night, she went to bed directly from the dinner table.

In November, she had another endoscopy. Given her symptoms, I was praying it would show a return of active disease. Maybe then, I hoped, her doctors would prescribe the magical "full dose." Instead, the doctor came into the recovery suite with pictures of a perfectly pink, smooth esophagus.

Dr. Dryfus, the younger doctor in the practice who had taken over Sammi's clinical appointments the year before, called us a few nights later to talk about the biopsy results.

"No eosinophils at all," he said. "Which is kind of amazing."

"It doesn't make sense," I said. "She's so sick!"

"I know," he responded. "I know. I really do. That's why I wondered if we might look at some other possibilities."

David and I locked eyes for a moment, listening on separate phones. For years, I'd been asking the gastroenterology team about "other possibilities."

"OK," David said on his extension. "What's the first possibility?"

"Well," the doctor began, "one concern I have is about Sammi's complaints that food 'comes back up.' Have you ever heard of rumination?"

"Isn't that what cows do? Chewing their cud?" I asked.

"It can be," he answered. "But it can also mean that the stomach muscles spasm, or release, and food shoots up the esophagus. It's something that happens in several populations—developmentally disabled people, people with a history of bulimia, etcetera. One thing I'm wondering is if Sammi has begun to do this subconsciously as a response to your anxiety—and her own—at mealtime."

"Anxiety?" I asked. "I'm not sure I understand."

"Well," he said, "you've mentioned that dinner is a stressful time for your family. It takes Sammi longer to eat than the rest of you, for example."

"That's definitely true," I said. "But what choice do we have? She has to eat."

"Well," he said, "she might feel a lot of pressure around that, if it's something she perceives as important to you."

"Important to *me*?" I asked, surprised. "It's important to *everyone*, every doctor we've ever seen. They all tell me I'm not feeding her enough. They all tell me she has 'failure to thrive.' We've even been threatened with feeding tubes. What am I supposed to do?"

"Mrs. Lewis," Dr. Dryfus said, "you absolutely cannot feed her enough to make her grow more than she already is."

I paused. "I'm not sure I understand."

"Sammi is congenitally small," he answered. "She's followed her growth curve, generally speaking, since birth. To give her enough calories to affect any change to that—even if it *is* a matter of calories—would require tube feeding. But she's not really a candidate for that. She's a little on the thin side, but not dangerously so."

"So no matter what I feed her, she's not really going to grow any faster?"

"No. You cannot do this through calories alone," he answered.

I could have wept. So much of our life together was focused on calories, density, volume, and quality—all the pressure heaped in each grocery bag, each soup pot. I wanted to take a moment to reconcile this history with this doctor's position, but there wasn't time.

"OK," I said, trying to absorb it all, "so you think, maybe, she's worked herself up at dinnertime—and all day long—and is subconsciously getting her stomach to propel everything back up to her throat?"

"It's possible," he answered. "Really, it can happen without thinking to anyone with stomach muscles that have been somehow conditioned to it."

"Sammi never throws up, though," I mused aloud. "She just says the food is coming up in her throat, but we never see it."

"Well, Sammi might actually always swallow before it can come out," he suggested. "It's a possibility that, for her, there's some kind of dysmotility involved—I actually consulted a friend of mine who is a specialist in dysmotility to see what he thought about Sammi's case."

"Oh, yes," I said. "That makes at least a little sense. There was some talk about her esophageal motility years ago, after the double aortic arch surgery."

There was a pause on the other end, and the doctor said, more slowly than before, "Really? Tell me about that."

"Well, it's probably all there in your records," I replied, "but they did dilate her esophagus at that time, after the surgery, and the GI doc who did the dilation mentioned that she might have some moderate dysmotility. That's probably in his report, though, right?"

"Well," Dr. Dryfus said quickly, "I mean, she has a long chart—really, really long—and I haven't had a chance to read the whole thing. . . ."

I looked up and across the dining room table, past the space between me and David, all the way to where he stood at the kitchen counter with a notepad and pen. He looked at me, his hand poised above the paper, and I made a panicked gesture. *How*, I telegraphed to him with wide eyes, *could he not have read Sammi's chart?*

"Where did she have the double aortic arch repaired then?" the doctor continued.

"Your hospital," I said quietly, feeling my body shift into automatic. In fact, I'd been answering questions like this for years, over the phone, with this same hospital. Before every endoscopy, the presurgical certification team would call me and ask the same dozen questions. *Is she on any blood thinners? Is she allergic to any medications? Has she ever had surgery before? Has she ever been followed by cardiology?* After the last question, I'd recite the history of Sammi's double aortic arch diagnosis and repair and insist we'd been released from care by all cardiologists and cardiothoracic specialists. Sometimes I'd need to call some of those doctors and verify information again, because presurgical screeners had different levels of trust in what parents said. The process was fairly straightforward because it could be done almost entirely electronically, the simple matter of a box ticked on a form.

"She had it repaired here?" the doctor responded. "OK, that's so interesting. That's really interesting, actually! Tell me about how you got that diagnosis in the first place. Was she having trouble breathing?"

My heart started to pound, my fingers went icy, and my armpits itched with cold sweat. He didn't know. He didn't know what had happened to Sammi when she was a baby—didn't know about the compression in her chest, didn't know how we'd plucked pouched blueberries out of her cheeks and then held her, cords everywhere, in the hospital room after a doctor had opened her back and seen the parts of her that we never would—her tiny heart, her one-year-old aorta. I dug my fingernails into my thighs to keep from panicking and told him the whole story: the respiratory infections, the reflux, the food refusal, the slow growth, the hospitalizations, the retracting chest and neck. When it was done, his voice filled with tangible excitement.

"This is so interesting," he repeated. "I wish I'd known about this before." There was a pause then, so pregnant a pause that it felt like it lasted seven years, the seven years between her aortic arch surgery and today. A flicker of memory passed behind my eyes of the times when I sat in an examining room with our first gastroenterologist—*Doctor, could this have anything to do with her double aortic arch?*—and heard only the sound of him tapping at the keyboard, his back dismissing my words before they even exited my mouth.

"OK, here's what I'm wondering," Dr. Dryfus finally said. "Sometimes, when there is dysmotility, food and acid can spend a lot more time in the esophagus instead of passing right through. They just kind of . . . sit there, rubbing up and down as the esophagus tries to move them through. That can cause some irritation."

"That makes sense," I said aloud, my teeth chattering as I came to realize what he was insinuating.

"Right!" he replied, getting even more excited. "And all that irritation can bring white blood cells to the surface to try to help."

"White blood cells . . . like eosinophils?" I asked.

"Exactly!" he replied. I could hear the smile in his voice and shuddered.

"Excuse me for interrupting, Doctor," David said from his extension, "but when Sammi was diagnosed with eosinophilic esophagitis, we were told that only reflux or EoE could bring eosinophils to the surface of the esophagus, and the numbers she had could be only from EoE. Has that conclusion changed? Because it sounds like you're saying that irritation can bring eosinophils into the picture."

"Well, of course it can!" the doctor said. "We're not always able to pinpoint the exact triggers for this irritation, which is why we do the diets and the meds and so on, but if this is a child with a history of dysmotility, we should look at that as a possible cause, for sure."

The call ended quickly after that, preceded by the doctor's enthusiastic plans for several tests and the sounds of Ronni and Sammi loudly nearing the end of their game of Uno upstairs. There wasn't time for

David and I to talk about the staggering revelation we'd just had before we tucked the girls into bed for the night, and when we came downstairs afterward, we found our dishwasher flooded with brown water. As I washed dishes in the bathroom sink and David bailed the dirty water out the back door, we vowed to talk about it the next day.

But the truth was that we never really talked about it. Instead, we acted on it, beginning with a series of medical tests for Sammi that would set us—finally—in motion toward a real, honest-to-goodness finish line. We threw our feelings about Sammi's unread chart and the doctor's half-explanation out the back door with the dirty dishwater. There was work to do.

7

MARSHMALLOW FLUFF
AND RASPBERRIES

Though David and I didn't talk about what the doctor had "discovered," after beginning the process of scheduling the first test, I turned to some of my closest friends to share what was happening.

While I waited for the radiology department to call me back, I began exchanging Facebook messages with Cathy, the friend who accompanied me to the hospital for Sammi's first surgical procedure all those years ago. I walked her through our conversation with the doctor, and her outrage matched mine.

"Pardon me while I stop banging my head on the desk," she typed, finally.

She came to understand the situation much as I had: no one in the gastroenterology practice had ever considered any previous structural issues in Sammi's chest that might account for her current symptoms. As I typed frenetically into my laptop, I could imagine Cathy on the other end, shaking her head. Eventually, she asked me what we were going to do.

"I think we need to get through these tests first and figure out a plan," I typed.

But, of course, I was livid. Later, I would learn that the information about Sammi's double aortic arch surgery was literally at the bottom of every surgical report in her record. At the time, though, I imagined it as something buried deep within. Still, my anger came out in a series of sarcastic messages in response to Cathy's question about how we might bring our concerns to the hospital:

"How about this?" I began, outlining a potential chart-reading protocol. "Has this patient had any procedures in the past that could have any impact on the diagnosis you just made?

"Has this patient ever had anyone's hands touch the internal organ you are attempting to assess?

"Are you perplexed by this child's lack of adherence to the general norms of the diagnosis you made? Have you checked their ★&%@ chart?

"*Does this not seem right to you?* Have you checked their ★&%@ chart?

"*Did you just tell your patient's parents that their child is giving you gray hair because her case is so weird?* Have you checked her ★&%@ chart?"

"What a bloody nightmare," Cathy finally wrote.

She was right. It was a nightmare I never imagined, not in my most paranoid fantasies about what was *really* wrong with Sammi. I imagined worsening symptoms. I wondered if she'd ever grow to adult size, if she'd suffer from vitamin deficiencies, if she'd end up in the emergency room with food trapped in her gullet. I'd mapped out all kinds of terrible imagined futures, but none of them included what was about to happen.

The first test Sammi had to undergo, the barium swallow study, was the easiest one. When she and I arrived at the hospital that November morning in 2013, by some strange stroke of luck, the radiologist assigned to us was the same one who had administered the test to Sammi in 2006; I remembered his booming voice. If he was still here, seven years later, I assumed he was a swallow study expert.

I told him I remembered him. "You did this same test on Sammi when she was just a year old," I said.

"So what's been going on?" he asked gruffly.

"Well, she was diagnosed with eosinophilic esophagitis a few years ago. . . ."

"Oh, yeah," he answered, rolling his eyes, "her and everyone else. That's the new thing."

My stomach dropped. Was this diagnosis *trendy*? I took a few deep breaths as Sammi came out of the changing room in a hospital gown.

A normal, healthy esophagus is a long, thick tube that runs from the throat to the stomach along the back of the body, with a gentle curve about two-thirds of the way down as it passes the heart. As Sammi good-naturedly drank the thick, chalky liquid from a straw while lying on the examining table, the X-ray machine passing over her transmitted images to a screen above us, clearly outlining the barium's route through her esophagus.

It was ghastly to watch. The path of the barium through her esophagus made it immediately apparent that something was wrong. It was shaped like a bolt of lightning.

Sammi, who was beginning to learn the Hebrew alphabet, looked at the screen, pointed, and said, "Mommy, it looks like a zayin!" She was right; the letter with a curve at the top and two gentle turns in its descender was the same shape as Sammi's esophagus. I looked at the radiologist with wide eyes, and he slowly shook his head.

"I want to try something else," he said, leaving the room. "You can sit up, honey."

Sammi sat up on the table and pointed at the cup of barium I was holding. "Do I have to keep drinking?" she asked cheerfully.

"I don't know," I admitted. "Let's see what the doctor says."

The radiologist came back in the room with a Styrofoam cup and a plastic spoon. "This is marshmallow fluff," he said to Sammi. "You ever eat marshmallow fluff?"

She shook her head.

"It's sweet, honey!" he exclaimed. "You just eat one spoonful and we're going to watch on the screen, OK?"

She nodded. I scooped up one spoonful and fed it to Sammi, and she laid back on the table. The machine hummed back on and we watched the spoonful-shaped blob of fluff make its way into her throat on the X-ray.

"OK, let's watch it go down," he said.

It reached the first jagged, ninety-degree turn in her esophagus, and then I watched in horror as it went back up an inch, back down, back up, back down, over and over again while Sammi lay there. After about thirty seconds, the radiologist told Sammi to sit up for a minute. We looked at a book together, my heart pounding in my chest, then he told her to lie back down.

The spoonful of marshmallow fluff was still in her esophagus, going up and down, nearing her throat several times. It had been two minutes.

"That's enough," I said finally. "Do you have what you need? Can we stop?"

He nodded. "OK, go get dressed, honey," he said to Sammi.

She scampered off the table and into the attached bathroom to change. Though he wasn't supposed to tell me anything, the radiologist looked at me, leaned his mouth close to my ear, and said, more quietly than he'd ever spoken before, "You have to call Dr. Backer."

"The heart surgeon?" I asked, aghast. "Why? Why would I call him?"

He pointed a thick, stubby finger at the first indentation in Sammi's esophagus, a dark spot between two curves, and said in a barked whisper, "That's her *aorta!*"

In a parallel universe, I crumpled to the ground, screaming, *no, no, not this again. . . .* But in this universe, I had an eight-year-old girl at my side a moment later, grinning, excited about the french fries I'd promised for the ride home. In this universe, I was alone with her—no one to ask to be with her for a moment while I collected myself, no one to echo the thoughts in my head, the questions, the million directions in which neurons were firing, the fight-or-flight hormones that had surged when the doctor said those three words.

That's her aorta.

Somehow, after snapping a photo of the screen, I got Sammi home from the hospital, the promised french fries in hand. A few days later, I got a phone call from the gastroenterologist. I was lucky enough to be at my friend Andrea's house, surrounded by a circle of women friends. I motioned for them to stay with me in the room.

"Did you see the picture of her barium swallow?" I asked him.

"Sure did," he answered. "Well, that was something, wasn't it?"

"Yes," I said. "It was really alarming for me."

"I can imagine," he answered quickly. "In any case, I think it would be beneficial to have Sammi go to speech therapy to learn diaphragmatic breathing."

He went on to explain that he still wondered if Sammi might have rumination syndrome—the learned behavior he'd described during our phone call a few weeks before, in which she might subconsciously force herself to regurgitate her food. Diaphragmatic breathing, he suggested, might help her learn to relax at mealtimes and keep her from regurgitating. He offered to refer us for six sessions with a therapist.

I took a deep breath before I answered. I'd spent the days between the barium swallow study and this phone call learning about esophageal dysmotility, about the interaction between a right aortic arch and the esophagus, about children who'd needed second and third cardiothoracic surgeries after their double aortic arch had been repaired. Nervously, I stood and gripped a nearby banister with my free hand.

"Doctor, am I understanding correctly that Sammi's aorta is pressing her esophagus into several right angles?" I asked.

"Yes," he admitted. "It sure looks like it is."

"So that's a structural problem, right?" I pressed him.

"That's true."

"So do you think that learning diaphragmatic breathing is likely to solve that structural problem? Will it move her aorta out of the way?" I could feel my voice rising. Andrea looked up from across the room.

"Well," he acknowledged, "no. No, it won't."

"*Well*," I answered, my hands shaking, "I don't think I'll do that, then. I don't think I'll take my daughter to six sessions of diaphragmatic breathing therapy that won't help her, since we've already put her through a dozen endoscopies that didn't really help her. I think I'll stop putting her through things that don't help."

I could hear his discomfort in the way he breathed. There was a pause and he coughed. Finally, with a more formal tone than he'd taken before, he said, "That seems logical."

"Great," I answered. "Now are you going to call Dr. Backer or should I?"

Another awkward pause preceded his response. "Who is that, now?" he asked me.

"The cardiothoracic surgeon!" I exploded. "The one who did Sammi's original repair for her double aortic arch!"

"And . . ." he asked, obviously pained, "where does he practice?"

"In your hospital!" I answered, exasperated.

"I can do it," he said quickly. "I'll take care of it."

Several years later, I would read the notes in Sammi's chart and tease out the meaning of each complicated medical term the radiologist had included in his report. "Moderate hold up of contrast" meant that, as we'd seen, the barium-spiked liquid and marshmallow fluff stayed in her esophagus after she swallowed. "Reverse peristalsis at the level of the right aortic arch" meant that the muscles of her esophagus near where her double aortic arch had been repaired were working in reverse, moving the contents of her esophagus up instead of down. And "focal buckling and mild narrowing of the lumen of the esophagus" meant that her esophageal walls were literally buckling in on themselves.

Though I didn't have that language in front of me in the weeks after the swallow study, I instinctively began to understand why Sammi had avoided so many of the foods she avoided and why she always drank so much water with dinner. Seeing the liquid go down the Z-shaped path of her esophagus helped me to picture her descriptions of eating yogurt. She'd always said that she liked it, but it was "too slimy" for her to swallow. Now I pictured it, a thick, viscous substance trying to make it past the right turns on the way to her stomach. I could imagine it sticking to the walls of her esophagus, creating bubbles of air as it backed up at the kinked spots. I imagined the taste of it as it backed all the way up to her throat, acidic and surprising, all while her mother stood anxiously by, hoping she would take another bite soon.

Then I pictured the dinner table, with bites of quiche or homemade pizza or vegetable potpie on her fork as she gestures, chatting, waiting patiently for the bite she swallowed five minutes ago to make it all the way down into her stomach, running to the kitchen for water to help it along. Every bite must take so long, I realized, that eating a full meal would naturally take an hour. Horrified with myself, I called Dr. Backer's office every day to see if he'd read the barium swallow results. When he finally did, he sent word through his advanced practice nurse that Sammi should come in right away for another test.

It was just two weeks after the barium swallow study when David, Sammi, and I found ourselves standing in the room in the children's hospital that held the enormous computed tomography (CT) machine. Dr. Backer had ordered a "CT scan with contrast," a test that would allow the radiologists and Dr. Backer to see exactly how blood was flowing through her aorta and around her esophagus. We'd been waiting in a pre-procedure room for more than an hour, an enormous IV needle painfully stuck in Sammi's arm. I'd climbed into the bed behind her, holding her wrist in my hand so that nothing jostled her arm as David showed her pictures on his phone and we both tried to distract her. With the endoscopies, she'd been asleep for IV placement. This time, she was awake and frightened. Once we got to the room with the CT machine, I carefully climbed out of the bed, balling up my scarf under Sammi's arm to keep it steady.

The CT room was an incongruous funhouse, the walls painted with a circus theme, clowns and popcorn carts and elephants dancing in a ring. In the middle was the CT machine, not pretty or decorated but serious, gray, and foreboding, a giant mechanized tube with a cold, smooth bed protruding from it, just the right shape for a child. David and I donned huge lead aprons and neckbands, covering us from below our chins to above our knees. Sammi shivered in a tiny, thin hospital gown printed with pictures of Tigger, as the technician slid her inside. Though I'd worn protective lead aprons before when I'd accompanied Sammi for chest X-rays as a baby, this was the first time I would wear one while she'd have radioactive material coursing through her veins. Knowing that was hard enough, but then a radiology technician came out of the glass booth on the far wall holding a plastic cup of amber liquid with a straw in it.

"You're Mom?" he asked.

I nodded and he identified the contents of the cup as a mixture of apple juice and a liquid called OmniPAQUE, which works to "light up" areas that radiologists want to see via computed tomography. It was already coursing through Sammi's veins via an IV, but they also wanted to see how OmniPAQUE would light up her esophagus while she swallowed. That wasn't easy, and it made the next twenty minutes deeply disturbing.

In the years that followed, this scene was metaphorically represented in my dreams by all kinds of high-stakes, nearly impossible scenarios: I would find myself holding Sammi by the strings of her hospital gown over a cliff while trying to send a crucial email to a client; I would attempt to get a doctor to read a test result on the platform of a commuter train without waking Sammi, asleep in my arms; I would watch as Sammi tried to eat fruit dangling from a tree in a windstorm without the use of her arms.

That day, Sammi, on her back, lay inside the CT machine, the IV bag hanging just outside the entrance to the tunnel. Because my arms were too short, David stood outside the machine with the cup and straw. As Sammi's heartbeat and the IV-borne OmniPAQUE pumped through her aorta, the radiology techs shouted through the room's speakers for Sammi to take a sip of the liquid in "three . . . two . . . one" and hold it in her mouth for "three . . . two . . . one" then swallow, timing it all to the rhythm of her heartbeat.

I stood there in my lead gown as my daughter's body pulsed with ionizing radiation and my husband's unprotected arm reached into the machine to give it to her. In a hospital as large and prominent as this one, I was in awe of the risks we were taking and—more importantly—of the way we were relying on the timed swallowing of an eight-year-old girl. I knew how long fluid stayed in her esophagus. I knew we were rubbing the inside of her esophagus with OmniPAQUE. And, in an incongruous moment of knee-jerk parenting, I wondered if Sammi thought this apple juice was a special treat; I never kept juice in the house.

As we waited for the results of the CT scan, the friends who knew what was happening began, tentatively, to ask if we were going to sue the gastroenterologist. Indeed, that had been my first instinct after our phone call with him, but as time wore on, I realized that the thought of it frightened me. I needed that doctor not to see me as an enemy. His office was just a few floors away from the surgeon's, and it was above our city's only children's hospital. The anger I felt was second only to my fear that no one would be able—or willing—to help us. I was afraid that if we started making public accusations against one doctor in this hospital, the hospital itself would refuse to help Sammi. My angry words to that gastroenterologist on the phone at Andrea's house haunted me at night. *He knows that I know,* I thought. *What will he do?*

Finally, though, Dr. Backer received the results from the CT scan and invited David and me to meet with him. A week before Sammi and Ronni's winter break, David and I dropped them off with Andrea and her family so that we could go to see Dr. Backer alone. In his office high above the cardiac ward of the hospital, he drew us a rough sketch of Sammi's thoracic anatomy on a sheet of notebook paper using red and blue pens to illustrate the flow of blood and to differentiate the major organs involved: heart, trachea, esophagus. Her aorta was crossing her esophagus from right to left at the same spot where her esophagus was zigzagging from left to right, trapped on one side by scar tissue from her previous surgery. The solution, he told us, was to move her aorta away from that part of her chest and over to the left side, where it ought to be, and then stitch it to the chest wall so it wouldn't be able to edge its way back.

He pulled up a series of files on his computer to show us the 3D images generated from the CT scan. Turning them left and right, rotating them with his mouse, he showed us models of our daughter's chest—organs and tissue he'd seen once with his own eyes and, if we agreed, that he would see again.

"It's pretty great that we can get these pictures now," he said. "Otherwise we do these procedures flying blind."

We asked him what would happen to Sammi if she didn't undergo this procedure. He looked thoughtfully up at the ceiling for a moment and then leaned his arms on the desk across from us. On the edge nearest me was a photograph of him with his family, children gathered around him. When he spoke, I could hear him weighing his words.

"Well, I suppose you could wait, if you wanted," he said, "but the esophagus, you know, it's a series of muscles. They're working in opposition to each other in Sammi, in a way, with some pushing to bring the food down and some in reverse. Eventually, they're going to wear out, working like this. They're already in a pattern that's not working very well for her."

As he went on to describe the alternatives down the line—removing a section of intestine to replace the esophagus when it gave out, for example—I thought about our own family patterns that were, without question, not working for us. I thought about dinner with our friends Christine and Jonathan and how their three kids all finished eating so much more quickly than Sammi that they had to sit, patiently but squirming, until she finished before they could all play together. I thought about beautiful summer nights when a family walk after dinner would have been fun if only Sammi could finish her meal before bedtime. I thought about how much my relationship with Sammi revolved around how much and what kind of food she ate, the exact reverse of the Weight Watchers guidance I watched during my childhood but probably, I realized, no less impactful.

Dr. Backer agreed to find a slot for the surgery during the week of her spring break. Before we left, he gave us a strongly worded warning about what foods were safe for her.

"Her normal diet is basically fine," he said. "But no meat. Really, absolutely none until she's had the surgery. It's very hard for her esophagus to get something that firm down, even if you cut it up very small."

"That's not a problem," I'd promised, smiling a little when I thought about my conversations with the pediatrician. "We're vegetarians."

"Well, this isn't the time to change that," he said. "Even a stuck bite of steak could get impacted, and with her aorta that close . . . and a chicken bone swallowed by accident would be really dangerous."

We said goodbye to him and walked to our car in the parking garage. Both of us were deeply shaken even though we had suspected Dr. Backer's news. It was a dark, cold night, and I sat shivering in the passenger seat as David drove us away from downtown Chicago and up Lake Shore Drive. I know we talked—we must have—but what I remembered years later about that night was how paralyzed I felt. I remember staring into my lap, shaking despite the car's heater, calling David's mom and my parents from the car. I remember trying not to cry as I whispered a shortened version of the plan to Andrea as the kids raced in and out of the room, laughing and playing.

Without having known we would need it, we had somehow packed the next week full of social gatherings with friends. We had Shabbat dinner with Christine and Jonathan and their children the next night, and when the kids were settled with an after-dinner movie, we told the adults what was happening. Christine's firm but kind insistence that we allow them to take care of us that night helped allay the creeping anxiety that had begun to settle in, at least for a few hours. The next night, we had plans with Ronni's best friend Zora's family, the ones who had always helped on the mornings of Sammi's endoscopies two years before. The day after that, we went to Milwaukee to visit old friends. It seemed that, just as the universe had sent the broken dishwasher to keep us from discussing the gastroenterologist's revelations in November, it was sending us a powerful reminder of the strength of our village now.

But eventually, reality did set in. Whenever David and I talked about it, alone in our bedroom before we went to sleep, one or both of us would be in tears. There was a lot to fear and even more to mourn. Much as I tried not to think about it, whenever I saw one of our old bags of gluten-free flour or rolled my grocery cart past the shelves of products on which we'd relied during the six-food elimination diet, a jolt of anger ripped through me, making my heart pound. If this surgery resolved Sammi's issues with eating, then we would know for sure that the year of the "joy-free diet" and all those endoscopies had been unnecessary. When I flashed back on all those times in the operating room, all the anxious meal preparation, and the dozen times I'd cried alone in my car in the grocery store parking lot, I experienced the same feeling I'd had listening to the gastroenterologist on the phone on the night of his big discovery: I began to sweat and shiver at the same time, my teeth chattered, and my hands shook.

I knew then that it was trauma I was feeling, coupled with a fury so keen that I fantasized weekly about trying to end the gastroenterologist's career once Sammi's surgery had been completed. My friend Amy indulged me in endless long walks during which I fumed and mused and worried. From coffee shop to coffee shop, she sat across from me and did her best to alternately distract and reassure, but I had read that, in broad numbers, roughly one in every 100,000 people who go under general anesthesia die. I found myself wondering whether that risk increased with every procedure. Was Sammi more at risk after the first five times? The first ten? Would the chance of death be higher this, her sixteenth, time? I told Amy that if Sammi died, I didn't know if we could stay friends; Amy's daughter Sophie was Sammi's best friend, and I didn't know if I could watch her grow up if Sammi remained forever eight. To her credit, Amy let me say it and then changed the subject.

In online chats with Hilary, who was living in Israel, she told me I seemed robotic. She offered to come for Sammi's surgery, but I told her to save her money for a trip when I'd be capable of enjoying her company. In the meantime, we shared recipes and talked about our work. Every so often, she'd try to convince me to let go of my commitments or seek therapy or even antianxiety medication, but I knew what I needed most: distraction. I helped bake for a friend who had to follow a special diet. I spent hours in my friend Rina's parents' house, helping her clean and pack her parents' antiques and collectibles for auction and donation. I took on more work, went for more and longer runs, and, as the days and weeks went on, allowed myself a few extra seconds to smell Sammi's freshly washed hair or run my fingers over her bare arms as we snuggled at bedtime.

As for food, it was a free-for-all. Aside from meat, which she didn't eat anyway, Sammi had no restrictions and—for the first time in her life—I no longer felt compelled to force-feed her. Still, I was in the habit of fixating on her diet, and in the absence of quantity, I became more obsessed with quality. Once I knew how much time solid food spent rubbing up and down in her esophagus, I refused to buy anything except organic produce. I didn't want harsh pesticides coating her gullet, so I spent a fortune on organic berries in particular, since they were the one food she really liked eating. When I sensed that she was well and truly frustrated after laboring over dinner each night, I simply offered her a bowl of raspberries.

"Even if I didn't finish my lentils?" she asked.

"Yes, it's fine." I told her, scrubbing a pot in the sink. "Go ahead."

If she was suspicious, she didn't say anything. With every bite she took, I pictured the spoonful of marshmallow fluff going up and down on the X-ray, retaining the shape of the spoon's cavity. I wondered how long every bite of pasta, every broccoli floret, every chunk of matzo ball took to finally reach her stomach. If raspberries, blueberries, and strawberries—and bowl after bowl of her favorite chickpea soup— somehow made their way past those kinks in her esophagus without hurting her, then I was going to feed them to her. Nothing else mattered to me anymore except making mealtime less stressful. For the last two years, I'd been asking, nudging, nagging, and sometimes angrily deriding her for not eating more quickly, when all along it wasn't that she *wouldn't* finish her dinner—it was that she *couldn't*.

The food had been *all the way to her mouth*. Now that I'd seen it, I couldn't ever forget.

About six weeks before the surgery, Dr. Backer's advanced practice nurse reached out to us to ask that we cancel any plans that included large gatherings or public places.

"If it was up to us, we'd tell you to pull her out of school for a month beforehand, but we know that's not really practical," she said. "I know you have an older child too."

Beginning exactly four weeks before the surgery, we surreptitiously began trying to prevent Sammi from getting sick and disqualifying herself for surgery. Her teacher, aware of the plan, had instituted extra hygiene practices in the classroom and sent a letter home to parents asking them to take extra care to keep students with sniffles out of school. I put hand sanitizer in Sammi's lunch box and asked her to use it after chorus practice and tae kwon do. Instead of attending our synagogue's fantastic Purim carnival—something all kids look forward to every year—we planned a carnival at my mother-in-law Susan's house, complete with crafts, fancy homemade chocolate-dipped strawberries, and a fingernail painting station. We told the kids it was because Susan missed us and we hadn't seen her in weeks. Susan, Sherri, Sherri's husband Rob, and David's Aunt Judy all joined us to make it more fun.

On the advice of the hospital social work team, our plan was to wait until about a week before the surgery to tell Ronni and Sammi. We'd bought a brand-new iPad that we hoped would be a distraction for both girls once we shared the news. As the day got closer and closer, it became harder to keep it from them.

Then, the night before we planned to tell the girls about the surgery, Ronni came down with a cold, putting all of our plans into jeopardy.

8

MATZO AND FAT-FREE
CREAM CHEESE

When Ronni came down with a bad cold nine days before Sammi's surgery, we panicked. On the advice of the hospital social workers, we hadn't even told them about the surgery yet. Based on the ages of the girls, the social work team had recommended we give them no more than a week's notice, but now we would have to tell them quickly so that they would understand why we had to separate them.

The conversation went surprisingly well, in no small part because we approached it as good news. We told them that we had figured out why Sammi's food came back up in her mouth, and the same doctor who had helped her when she was a baby was going to help us with this, too. When they found out how long she'd be in the hospital—six days at least—they were both upset until we showered them with exciting distractions: the iPad, a Netflix account, and the promise of a two-day sleepover at Christine and Jonathan's house for Ronni. They scampered off into the living room to play with the iPad, promising to wipe it off with disinfecting wipes between turns and sit a few feet apart to play.

For the rest of that day, we fed them in separate rooms and assigned them different bathrooms. I'd disinfected every doorknob and staircase railing before they woke up. Still, we thought, maybe there is something else—should Sammi take antibiotics and antivirals just in case? Should we have them sleep on different floors of the house? Should we open all the windows at night to let the germs out? We called the advance practice nurse in Dr. Backer's office later that day.

"The best thing you can do," the nurse told us, "is get Sammi out of there."

With tears in my eyes, I packed a bag of clothes and other necessities for Sammi, picked her up from school on Thursday, and drove her to Susan's house. Early in the morning, for the last day of school before break, she drove Sammi the forty-five minutes to school and back again to her house to sleep that night. All Friday night, I sat on the opposite end of the couch from Ronni and watched Harry Potter movies with her while Sammi snuggled with her grandmother, safely far away.

In the end, Sammi stayed away from home for four days. On the second night, I tried to sleep at my mother-in-law's house to be closer to her, but I couldn't settle down—I laid in bed reading and playing games on my phone, constantly worried, listening to my heart beat hard against the mattress whenever I lay down. The next night, I went home and watched basketball on the other side of the couch from Ronni again, leaning against David's back. I made Ronni elaborate meal trays with her favorite foods, tiny vases of flowers, and pretty arrangements of cookies, eager to minister to her while desperate not to get sick myself. The idea of being kept away from the hospital while Sammi was there made my stomach drop into my feet.

Eventually, though, Ronni's cold got better, and Sammi came home to spend the last few days before surgery at home, since it was the beginning of her spring break. We went on hikes and played at the park, downloaded movies to the iPad, and baked chocolate-mint cupcakes for no reason except that we wanted them. I wasn't even trying to tempt her with foods that would pack on extra pounds before surgery; I just wanted us to enjoy ourselves.

On the day of the surgery, we woke early and packed the bags of books, clothes, and snacks into the car, bringing Sammi and Ronni out last so that they could stumble out of bed and into the car in their pajamas. The night before, as I'd tucked Ronni into bed, she'd asked me a question with tears in her eyes.

"Momma," she asked, one hand twisting my hair around her finger like she'd done since she was a baby, "could Sammi die tomorrow?"

"I was worried about that, too, sweetie," I explained, squeezing her free hand. "But last week, I called Dr. Backer and asked him what the chances of that were."

"You did?" she said, eyes widening.

"Yes. He said that he can never tell anyone that the chances of a patient dying in surgery are zero, but this surgery isn't very dangerous. He said he has never seen anyone die during this surgery. Not ever."

"Really?" she asked.

"Really," I told her, wrapping my arms around her and burying my face in her lush curly hair.

"Thank you, Momma," she whispered in my ear.

I wasn't lying. My fear had started to bring me, in the middle of the night, to Sammi's room, where I would stand by her bed and watch her sleep, trying to memorize her face and her hair and the way she slept with one knee up, her foot flat on the bed. I was hugging her too tightly and for too long. It was too hard to sit with my fear without knowing, so I called Dr. Backer one day and asked him directly what the odds of her dying might be.

He'd told me what I later told Ronni and put Sammi's chances of death around 1 to 2 percent.

"There are other complications, though, that I was going to tell you about when we talked right before the surgery," he went on, "but I can tell you a little about them now, if you want."

"Please do," I told him. "I'd rather know it all and be able to prepare."

"Well, the most common complication is that we bump her vocal cords during intubation or during the bronchoscopy Dr. Holinger is going to do," he started. "If that happens, she might have some changes to her voice, but it's usually temporary.

"The second most common complication is that we nick one of her thoracic ducts while we're moving her aorta or her esophagus. Those ducts are tiny veinlike threads that move dietary fat through the body. If we nick one of those, she might need to stay a little longer in the hospital after the surgery until we're sure it's healed, and she might need to change her diet a little during that time. We'll let you know if that happens."

"Diet changes are no big deal to us," I said. "We've done plenty of that."

"Good, good," Dr. Backer continued. "The more major complications have to do with her esophagus. If it's accidently punctured, then healing can be much more complicated, and we might even need to postpone completing the operation. It's unlikely, but it's possible."

The rest of the complications he described were the ones common to any surgery: issues with anesthesia, breathing tubes, and blood pressure, all likely to be expertly managed by the anesthesiologist.

"Does that cover your question?" Dr. Backer asked, finally. "I don't want you to go into this feeling like you don't know something you want to know."

"No, thanks, Doctor," I answered him. "It just seemed like there were so many more lethal possibilities in a surgery like this. I needed to know."

"No problem, Mrs. Lewis," he replied. "This is a big deal to your family, but it's one of the least complicated procedures I do. I promise you—I feel good about Sammi's prognosis. I really do."

Knowing that was helpful, but it didn't change the irrational part of me that had looked at the new loft bed we'd bought Sammi that spring and thought to myself that it was going to be a huge pain to get it out of the house if she died. It was maudlin, but it was real. Everything I could plan by then had been planned—her return to school with accommodations for her recovery, her bag packed with the pajama bottoms she liked, her hair freshly washed and set in tight braids I hoped would last her entire hospital stay—so all that was left to do with my nervous, anxious heart was to plan what I would do if she died.

Fortunately, I had brought one thing with me that day just for me: my friend Rebecca. Her daughter Celia and Sammi were very good friends at the time, and when Rebecca had asked how she could help, I'd asked if she would spend the day at the hospital with us. I knew that David's mother, sister, and brother-in-law would be there, but they felt like supports for Sammi and David. They were generous and kind and supportive of me in all ways, but with my parents so far away and my brother busy with his work and his young children, I wanted someone to stand in for my own family. Rebecca was calm, warm, and steady, and she fit right in with David's family, too.

Much of the surgery day routine was familiar to us from our many endoscopies but with one variable: instead of the normal surgery floor and waiting room, I walked Sammi into the cardiac theater, a much larger operating room with far more equipment. Years later, I would read the beautiful book *Counting Backwards* by Henry Przbylo, one of the anesthesiologists at the hospital where Sammi had this surgery. He wrote about his position at the head of the operating table during surgeries as a command center for all the patient's bodily functions, a sacred space where he watched carefully to ensure not one heartbeat or breath changed that wasn't part of the surgeon's plan. To Dr. P, as he liked to be called, this was where his brain went into hyperfocus, making him one of the most frequently requested anesthesiologists in the hospital.

For me, though, this room was new. I hadn't been allowed in the operating room for Sammi's first cardiac procedure—I had begun insisting on it after that—and so the differences were notable and overwhelming. Sammi noticed them, too, asking me why this room was different, what that device was, how long I was going to stay. As the nurses scooped her from the gurney to lay her on the operating table, her eyes widened.

"It's warm!" she exclaimed. "And squishy!"

The nearest nurse's eyes smiled above her mask. "It's your very own waterbed," she explained. "To keep you toasty warm while the doctor takes a look at you."

"Is it a *water* bed or a *matzo ball soup* bed?" I whispered in Sammi's ear. She giggled when I added, even more quietly, "Well, it's Passover this week. It might just be matzo balls!"

In truth, the warm waterbed mattress was there to prevent hypothermia in the cold operating room, where she would lie facedown on the table, her entire back and legs bared for the surgeon once she was fully anesthetized and her insides open to the cold air. Instead of telling her that, we proceeded as we always had, with the strawberry-scented gas, the song, the kiss on her forehead, and my horrible walk down the hall and ride up the elevator to where David and his family and Rebecca were waiting, this time in a beautiful, bright waiting room on the cardiac floor of the hospital.

It was a long, terrible morning and early afternoon. At one point, Sherri offered to pick up lunch, and I couldn't think of anything I wanted to eat. Just as Susan caught me looking worried and repeated, several times, "Debi, she's going to be just fine," Sherri put her hand on my arm and told me, firmly, that I would be no good to Sammi if I didn't take care of myself. It seemed like only a moment later that a gorgeous, bountiful salad from one of my favorite downtown restaurants appeared in front of me.

Time warped and stretched until the moment that Dr. Backer's nurse came out, three hours and twenty minutes after I walked out of the operating room with Sammi's damp forehead imprinted on my lips. I didn't know how to feel; the procedure had been scheduled to take six hours in total. If she was done in half that time, was it good news or bad news?

"She did great," the nurse told us. "Dr. Backer will be out to explain more in a few minutes. They're closing now."

Closing meant that they were closing the incision, closing my daughter's body back up. For about fifteen minutes, then, we were in a kind of nowhere land, knowing Sammi was OK but not knowing what exactly had happened. When Dr. Backer came in the room, we all stood up as though he were a head of state.

"Everything went perfectly," he said immediately. "We did the whole thing through one incision, right through her old scar."

"Wow, really?" I asked, incredulous. He had told us he'd likely need to make two incisions, one on each shoulder blade. "You could do it all from the left? Did you think you could do that before?"

"Well, I thought we might," he admitted, "but I wasn't sure, and I didn't want to get your hopes up. Anyway, we moved her aorta out of the way and pexied it to her chest wall, which is very secure and not going to go anywhere . . ."

"That's great," Susan said.

". . . and then we cleaned up a surprising amount of scar tissue. It's probably from her first surgery. It was . . . well, a lot of it, all around her esophagus. It was stuck on the other side, opposite her aorta. The area was weeping pretty badly, so we've left a drain tube in there. We'll keep an eye on it. There's a good chance we nicked one of those thoracic ducts I mentioned before. She'll be on fat-free food for a few days at least. Let's just see."

"Such good news, Doctor," David said, standing to shake his hand.

"I'm glad too," Dr. Backer said. "My nurse will let you know when you can go see her. She did great."

As soon as Dr. Backer was out of the room, David turned, buried his face in my neck, and burst into tears. Susan, Sherri, Rob, and Rebecca walked to the other side of the room to give us some privacy, and

I held David as he sobbed. I could feel all the emotion he'd been holding in vibrating against my chest.

To my surprise, I wasn't feeling anything.

I expected to cry, to release, to feel relief, but all I could find when I dug for feelings was a wary sort of curiosity. Even with the surgeon declaring success, there was still so much potential for disaster.

I had read that it was not uncommon for parents to experience dissociation in the twenty-four hours after their child has an operation. The feeling of being both there and elsewhere—aware of the risk and the fear but living outside it—is an expedient coping mechanism, and I was leaning on it hard. If my behavior all those times I'd been in the operating room felt like a pantomime, finding a way to manage this rush of David's feelings while mine were absent almost felt like playing a video game. *I should rub David's back a little*, I thought, and I made my arms move, and I kissed the side of his head, and I waited, my eyes clear.

A few minutes later, a nurse from the cardiac intensive care unit came to offer us a chance to bring our things to Sammi's room before she was wheeled up. Grateful for something to do, I went in and arranged her stuffed animals and dolls on the shelf opposite her bed, photos of her friends in front of them, and our family photo album open to a picture of Ronni in the center. I left our bags in the corner on an upholstered window seat that would later convert into a bed and went back out to the waiting room to rejoin our group.

By now, I'd sent an update message to everyone and posted on Facebook, and responses were steadily coming in. The deluge of "such good news!" "wonderful—keep us posted" "*baruch hashem* (bless G-d)" and "so glad to hear" felt like too much for me. There was a small, angry voice I kept hearing in my head that said *suckers. This isn't over. It's never over.*

Finally, though, a nurse told us Sammi was ready for us to come see her. Only two people were allowed in her room at a time, so David and I went first.

She was propped up a little in her bed, her eyes fluttering. She was holding an on-demand morphine pump button in her right hand, and one of her braids had come entirely undone. There were tubes and wires everywhere. We approached the bed and each kissed her face, and she opened her eyes.

"It's all done, Sunshine," I told her. "You did everything you needed to do, and now you just get to start feeling better."

"We love you so much," whispered David.

I smoothed the hair off her face and asked if there was anything she needed.

Water, she mouthed, her eyes half-closed.

"Is that OK?" I asked the nurse, who nodded and left to get a cup with a straw. When she returned, we held the straw to Sammi's lips. She took a small sip, and as she swallowed, her eyes widened.

"Does it hurt?" I asked.

She shook her head and mouthed *cold*. Her throat was clearly raw from more than three hours of intubation, a rigid plastic piece holding her airway open through the deep sleep of anesthesia.

After everyone else had taken a turn to visit with her, the long, slow rhythm of hospital time began. To recall a full day during that recovery would be dull: vital signs checked every hour, two hours, four hours, X-ray technicians who wheeled their machines into the room every morning at 5:00, balloons and teddy bears that arrived from the gift shop. The clock ticked, the room stayed quiet, and Sammi requested movies and instantly fell asleep once they began.

The one new thing was the chest tube. It was the most present, visceral reminder of what actually had happened to Sammi in the operating room. Out of an opening in the side of her chest behind her left armpit came a rubber tube, flexible and narrower than a drinking straw. At the end of the tube was a round rubber bulb that filled, day and night, with the loose contents of her chest cavity. The fluid inside the bulb was mostly pink with occasional clear stripes. It was the result of what Dr. Backer had called "weeping," a byproduct of the removal of all that scar tissue and the damage done to one thoracic duct. The fluid was partially dietary fat leaking out of the damaged duct. Several times a day, a nurse emptied the bulb, but not before doing something they called "milking" it.

The nurse squeezed the top of the tube, close to the opening in Sammi's chest, and ran her fingers down its length, pulling the fluid into the bulb. Sammi said it hurt, and I assume that was the result of the tug against the two stitches that held the tube in place. It was a surreal thing to watch, made more distressing when it called to mind memories of pumping breast milk for her and Ronni. I had pulled and tugged at my breasts in the service of nourishment. Now I watched the nurses use the same motions to give Sammi more space to breathe, draining the fluid pooling around her lungs.

"I'll hold your hand, OK?" I told her, rushing to the opposite side of the bed each time. She sometimes reached out a hand, trailing an IV behind her, and sometimes shook her head slowly, preferring to stay focused inward for the minute or two it took.

To keep the bulb from pulling her stitches when she moved, the nurses put a safety pin through a plastic tab on its side and pinned it to Sammi's hospital gown. I hated looking at it, the open end of a wound I'd not only allowed someone to inflict on her but *requested*. Every time they milked her tube, she whimpered and I ached.

At eight o'clock the first night, her nurse suggested she try to eat something. I was surprised—it seemed so soon—but she said it was worth trying. Because Sammi had suffered the surgical complication we'd been warned about—chylothorax—she'd been ordered to eat a fat-free diet for now. To our surprise, the on-demand hospital food service had a fat-free menu. I sat on the edge of Sammi's bed and read her some choices.

All she wanted was strawberries and some juice. When they arrived, we propped her up in bed. For the tenth time in four hours, I wanted to rebraid her hair, but instead I tucked it back behind her ear.

"Do you want to do it, or should I feed you?" I asked.

"I can do it," she said, her voice a crackly whisper. She picked up the fork, IV tubes dangling and tangling with each other as she speared a strawberry. For the second time that day, she swallowed and opened her eyes wide, surprised.

"You look like that felt funny," I noted. "Does it hurt? Or feel weird?"

"It feels different," she said, her voice a little stronger.

"How?" David asked her, rubbing her ankle under the blankets.

"It feels different with the food going down. It's not like *chkk chkk chkk*, it's like *ssssshhhhhuwwww* really fast," she said and leaned back into her pillows to swallow another berry.

David and I looked at each other, and my eyes finally filled with tears. *It worked*, I mouthed.

The first two nights, I slept at the hospital with Sammi and David went home to sleep. After that, we took turns going home to Ronni, whose soul hurt every bit as much as Sammi's due to their separation. Ronni was a few years too young to visit Sammi, so they relied on Face-Time whenever Sammi was awake enough to talk. Nights home with Ronni were delicious; we got takeout dinner one night, and another night went to Christine and Jonathan's house for a very short Passover seder (the traditional religious service over a ritual meal) with them.

The nights in the hospital seemed an entirely different world. The first two nights, getting Sammi adequate pain relief was a challenge as we waited to hear from the gastroenterology team about whether a particular kind of pain medication recommended by the palliative care team was safe for Sammi, considering the status of her gastroesophageal reflux. For an entire night, I asked the nurse over and over whether anyone had heard from them, but they never responded. At one point during the evening, Sammi was in so much pain that she stared me in the eyes and screamed, "Why am I being punished?"

The next morning, I was waiting outside the room when the pain team made their rounds. "Give her the medicine," I told them. "We'll deal with her reflux if it bothers her." In the end, we never heard from the gastroenterology team—not then and not ever again.

Once the issue of her pain medication was resolved, though, we had hours of time during which Sammi was in a kind of drugged haze, awake but not enough to play cards or color or play with any of the cool toys Susan had brought her. Instead, I turned on her favorite movies, over and over, until she fell asleep again or until her latest food tray arrived.

Sammi was definitely going to stay on a fat-free diet for a while, they told me, though the doctors mostly avoided the question of "how long" when I asked. She was allowed to order anything she liked off the à la carte menu, and she delighted in my willingness to let her decide all on her own. With every meal, she ordered either a Sprite or a bright blue Powerade, a bowl of strawberries, and an Italian ice. Though she had done well with the fat-free macaroni and cheese and the bowl of corn, she was still leaning toward wet, sweet, and cold.

The one time I pushed her was the second night of Passover. When David and I explained to Sammi that I would go with Ronni to a seder at Christine and Jonathan's and he would go with Ronni to the next seder at Amy and Ben's, her response was, "What about Passover for me?"

Her words filled me with a longing and sadness that took me by surprise. Any other year, I'd be hosting a seder myself. By this time the year before, I'd already spent days shopping for ingredients, wine, and fancy paper plates since our guest list had long ago outgrown our china settings. I had planned the seder itself for weeks beforehand, finding interesting new readings to intersperse throughout, copying slips of paper for everyone to fill out with what they were grateful for that year. The morning of the seder, Ronni and Sammi took their usual positions on the kitchen floor with boxes of matzo, crushing each sheet into pieces for our family's favorite matzo stuffing. I'd chopped until my arm hurt: carrots, onions, celery, and garlic, all to mix with the matzo crumbs, eggs, seasonings, and margarine, which we wrapped in tinfoil to bake in the oven later. I made dozens of matzo balls in that comforting broth with vegetables that Sammi had always loved and then began chopping ingredients for charoset, a salad of apples, nuts, cinnamon, and wine meant to represent the mortar in the bricks of the pyramids. There was lemon and sesame tofu for the main course, plus all of the rituals that a seder required: arranging hard-boiled eggs, chopped fresh parsley, horseradish, romaine lettuce, and the charoset on special "seder plates" designed for displaying them. It was a holiday that required a lot of preparation, and I was proud to have been up for it almost every year since David and I were married, beginning when I could barely cook at all until the year before, when we'd had more than twenty guests.

But this year, instead, I sat next to a hospital bed where my sad, tired, hurting daughter barely even knew what day it was. Fortunately, David's Aunt Maxine and Uncle Fred had called from the grocery store earlier in the day to ask if we wanted anything before they came to visit. I'd asked for a box of matzo and a jar of jelly so that Sammi and I could mark the day, at least in a small way. Around 7:00 at night, after we'd already FaceTimed with everyone at the seder, I stopped the movie Sammi was watching and pulled my chair up to the side of the bed.

"All right," I said. "We're going to have a seder."

She looked at me and said slowly, "OK?"

I stood up and pulled the grocery bag Maxine had handed me earlier in the day. I was closest with her of all of David's family members. With my parents and her son far away, we each fulfilled a need for the other, and she was the only one in the family who'd regularly asked me out to lunch, just the two of us. We had a great time together, too, and when she called from the grocery store, I felt seen. She hadn't just asked if there was anything *Sammi* wanted—she'd asked about me, too. She'd handed me the bag earlier and said, "I know you said just grape jelly, but I got you strawberry, too. You're like me; later you'll wish you had *options.*" Of course, she was right.

Taking the matzo and the jam out later that night, I asked Sammi if she remembered the most important things we had to discuss at a Passover seder. I put a slice of fat-free cheese from the hospital on a piece of matzo, handed it to her, and we talked about the story of the exodus from Egypt. As we chatted, a nurse came in and asked us what we were eating, and Sammi got the chance to tell her all about matzo. After that, I gave her a little piece of matzo with grape jelly on it and reminded her that even when times are hard, we can always find a little sweetness. I could see that even this short conversation was wearing her out, so I put away all the matzo and put on the movie *The Prince of Egypt*, an adaptation of the Passover story. In our own way, we'd had a seder. As I watched Sammi's eyes flutter closed, I felt more at peace than I had in the last few days.

The next afternoon, when David came to trade places with me, I took home the packet of information about chylothorax that Dr. Backer's team had given me that morning. Because of that small nick in one of her thoracic ducts, Sammi would need to stay on a fat-free diet for six weeks. At first, I'd thought it would be irritating but mostly not a big deal. I vaguely remembered how much food was fat free in the 1990s, when it seemed that half my friends were trying to eat as little fat as possible. I felt confident that I'd dealt with more difficult diets than this one.

Just to be sure, though, after I dropped Ronni off at school the next morning, I snuck into the grocery store for a few minutes on my way back to the hospital. Sammi's allotment of fat was 0.5 grams per meal. Thinking through what Sammi typically ate in a day, I began with breakfast. I started by looking for fat-free soy milk, which would be more like what she was used to drinking, and found one brand, way on the bottom shelf and nearly out of sight. Cereal posed more of a problem; her favorite cereal was 1.5 grams of fat per serving. The same was true for her next favorite, and on down the list. Even plain crisp rice cereal had 0.7 grams per serving. The only cereal I found that would work was definitely not going to be fun for Sammi. *That's OK,* I thought, *we'll let her put sugar on it.*

Moving through the store, I checked on some other favorites. Chickpeas were too high in fat. Plain pasta was too high in fat. Edamame was too high in fat. Tofu was way too high in fat. I kept looking at her favorites and feeling that familiar sense of dread I experienced grocery shopping for the six-food elimination diet; everything was a great big *no.* Even air-popped popcorn had a full gram of fat per serving. In a panic, I paid for my container of fat-free soy milk and several cartons of strawberries and reeled my way out of the store.

This diet was going to be the worst yet.

9

STRAWBERRIES AND SUSHI
AND MAKING DO

When we brought Sammi home from the hospital after a week in the cardiac unit, the challenges that faced us were both wildly different from what we'd encountered before and heartbreakingly similar. For the better part of eight years, we now knew, she'd never swallowed like a normal person does. Now it was up to us to teach her that she could, to remind her of the way her esophagus now moved in a straight line for the first time. Regardless of her newfound ability, though, I was looking once again at a diminished version of Sammi—this time, not just clinically measured in the pounds she'd lost in the hospital but obviously visible to everyone in her drawn face and her tiny slumped shoulders.

The day we brought her home—along with a trunk full of balloons and stuffed animals—Ronni had prepared a nest on the couch for her lined with down comforters and pillows and with important items strategically placed nearby, like tissues and a water bottle. On the wall across from the couch was a poster board that Ronni had carried from her middle school to the elementary school, clutching a handful of markers. She'd had all of Sammi's friends and favorite teachers sign it. "Welcome home, Sammi" and "you rock!" and "get well soon" and, over and over again, "we miss you" studded the poster. Even Ronni's friends had signed.

"I just wanted to *do* something," she'd told me when she'd shown me the day before. "Christine got me the poster board."

Ronni had spent the first three days when Sammi was in the hospital with Christine and Jonathan and their children, who had distracted her and kept her fed and loved and held while we worried over Sammi. That week I'd told Ronni that when Sammi came home, she was going to have to eat a fat-free diet for at least a month.

"That's OK," Ronni had said, squaring her shoulders, "we've done diets before."

"Right," I'd cautioned, "but this one is weirder and way harder, and we can't really all stay on it with her."

I went on to explain to her what had happened, the tiny duct in Sammi's chest nicked by a scalpel, leaking chyle into her chest cavity. "That chyle is the stuff that helps her body process fat in her food. It's still leaking, so she can't have any fat at all. It's a really big deal if she does," I explained. "She can't have even a little."

Ronni nodded. I could see her realization that this was different from the six-food elimination diet of Sammi's kindergarten year, even if she couldn't remember it as well.

"But this diet?" I'd gone on. "It's not healthy for people. It's only for Sammi, this time, and only for six weeks. You and me and Daddy have to go on eating regular food, but just—kind of carefully around her. Not exactly secretly, but not, like, in her face about it. Does that make sense?"

"Yeah," Ronni said. "So, what's she going to eat?"

That was a very good question. I'd begun to research fat-free food when we were in the hospital during that one quick trip to the store. The options were bleak and unappetizing, mostly. I'd felt that familiar sense of dread as I'd walked the aisles, reading the packaging once again. The nutritionist had told us that Sammi could have no more than half a gram of fat per meal. Standing in the frozen food aisle the day after Sammi came home, I called the nutritionist.

"I'm standing in the frozen section of the grocery store," I said, "and frozen corn looks like it has a gram of fat per serving."

She paused on the other end. "Well, does it have a sauce or something?"

I rolled my eyes. *I'm not an amateur*, I thought to myself. "No. It's just corn. That's the only ingredient."

She *hmmmed*, paused again, and said, "Well, she can only have foods that have half a gram or less of fat."

"I know," I said. "I read that and I understand. But she does love corn. Is there a brand you recommend that *does* have only half a gram per serving? You know, whatever you found that you put on this list you gave me?"

"No, sorry," she said.

"So, um," I paused, trying not to let the anger bubbling up inside me ooze through the phone, "how do I know which items on your list are really OK, then? Just read the labels?"

"Yes, you're going to have to be very careful with labels," she told me.

"I can do that," I said. "Really, this isn't our first experience with a limited diet. But then, should you take corn off the list for the next kid, maybe?"

"Well, as long as the corn has half a gram or less in it, it's fine," she said, a little more tensely now.

"But it doesn't," I pressed. "All the frozen corn in this store has a gram of fat per serving."

"Then that's not an item your daughter can eat," she answered firmly.

Dejected, I walked out of the grocery store that first day with almost nothing.

But even harder than the crummy culinary life I had ahead of me at my usual station at the stove was the knowledge that, once again, no one could help me. Before the surgery, when we'd thought she'd be coming home on an unrestricted diet, Amy had set up a meal train for us, bursting with people ready to bring casseroles and pots of soup and batches of muffins. We'd written to her from the hospital to cancel it all. We couldn't take meals from outside, not now; if anyone forgot the restrictions and sautéed the onions for their soup in olive oil, Sammi's chest might fill with chyle and drown her from the inside.

Instead, we asked Amy to have friends sign up to bring us washed, cut fruit. Once again, Sammi was going to enjoy an all-you-can-eat fruit buffet and thank heavens for it. Every other day, someone would ring my doorbell and hand over a gallon bag of perfectly cubed watermelon or a quart of glistening, trimmed whole strawberries. I watched nervously from the corridor outside the living room as Sammi held a single chunk of melon to her lips and sucked, pulling the juice from the fruit into her mouth. One cube of melon might last several minutes. Eating a bowl of it might consume an hour as she drowsily watched *Despicable Me 2* for the fortieth time.

That first day, though, all that was ahead of us as we set Sammi down gingerly in the nest in the corner of the couch, an area we called the "sweet spot." From the sweet spot, there were the supportive, tall edges of the couch backing her on two sides, and Sammi could alternate stretching her legs in both directions. I brought a little tray to her with a bowl of fresh blueberries, a tiny vase with a flower, and a cup with a straw, full of the horrible blue sports drink with which she'd been obsessed in the hospital. I was so afraid she'd stop drinking—crucial for clearing the fluid from her chest and for balancing the diuretic drugs she was taking—that I'd raced away from her and David on our way out of the hospital and bought three bottles of it in the cafeteria, shoved deep in my backpack as I waited at the door for David to bring the car around.

"Welcome to Momma's Restaurant!" I announced cheerily, setting the tray on the table in front of her. "Would you like some of my best Smurf Essence?" Sammi giggled at my name for her sports drink and nodded.

I watched her puff her cheeks out again as she swallowed and brushed my fingers against them. "You don't have to hold it in your mouth anymore, sweetie," I told her softly. "It's going to go down fast now, remember?"

"I know," she sighed. "Can I watch *Aladdin*?"

Thus it began. We tried to follow the same path that we had with the six-food elimination diet, choosing recipes that sounded good and rating them as a family, but this time, almost everything was unsatisfying. Fat, I had intuited but now was learning firsthand, transfers flavor through food more efficiently than any other ingredient. It makes food *look* better, provides a better mouthfeel, and, most importantly, contributes more than anything else to our sense of satiety—of feeling *full*. Without fat in our food, we are left feeling very, very unsatisfied.

In some instances, David, Ronni, and I tried to eat as Sammi did—cooking our vegetables in vegetable broth and eating the one tasteless brand of fat-free pasta we could find along with a fat-free tomato sauce. But the chylothorax diet, as it's known clinically, is required only when the injury to a thoracic duct is certain, like it was for Sammi, so I felt less guilt about not imposing this diet on the rest of us, for whom it was not only unnecessary but likely harmful. Ronni and David quietly added fresh parmesan to their pasta, and I continued to use our usual full-fat soy milk for me and Ronni in the mornings, pouring the nearly gray fat-free soy milk into Sammi's cereal bowl. I sent Ronni to friends' houses often during those weeks so she could get pizza or macaroni and cheese or fresh, warm cookies; I snuck outside and gobbled handfuls of cashews.

On Facebook and in emails to family, I asked for fat-free recipes and was hit with a deluge of Weight Watchers recipes I recalled from my mother's years of membership in the 1980s and 1990s: spaghetti squash and cabbage soup and salads dressed with vinegar, none of which were remotely attractive to Sammi. I tried a few, noting that the baked apple fritters we'd made with fat-free soy milk and egg whites would have been delicious if only they'd been fried.

On the six-food elimination diet, I'd recognized the things we ate as real food—if not the kinds of foods we'd eaten before, at least as the foods that other people ate. We'd learned about Indian popadums made of lentil flour; fried cornmeal masa cakes from Mexico called *picaditas*; miso paste from Japan that dissolved into flavorful broths. We'd found ways to use garbanzo flour for flatbread and to thicken vegan cream sauces made with nutritional yeast. We'd attempted to bread and deep-fry everything from bananas and red peppers to little vegetable dumplings we bought at the Korean grocery store. Our palates broadened, becoming more daring. I thought we could find things to love within the confines of any diet, but I was wrong.

On this diet, I dreaded making dinner every night. There were no lovely surprises in the world of 100-percent fat-free cooking. Meals became monochrome—if not in color, in mood—a drudgery of plain vegetables, egg whites, and lentils, every serving dish speckled at the bottom with seasonings that didn't stick to the food. Sammi barely picked at everything, perking up, as usual, only for fruit or the endless batches of meringues I made with egg whites and raspberry jello or cocoa powder. Nothing satisfied us; everything was a disappointment.

What was worse, a lot of the food I was buying barely qualified as food at all. It ran antithetical to all my lessons about what constituted healthy food before. When the kids had asked for Cheetos, which were one of the few foods I categorically refused to buy, my response was always, "that's not food; it's a science project." During the six weeks of Sammi's fat-free diet, though, we were swimming in science projects masquerading as food.

First, there were the fat-free versions of dairy products. The fat-free soy milk was really just watered-down regular soy milk, so that was tolerable, but the fat-free butter spray was utterly disgusting. Lactose intolerance be damned, I tried a little, not wanting to feed Sammi something I hadn't tested. It tasted like butter flavor and cheap lip balm, a strange oily sensation that then evaporated like alcohol. It came in a spray bottle, like glass cleaner, and when I sprayed it onto the fat-free bread I'd toasted, it soaked in immediately, staining the toast bright yellow. I shuddered.

The fat-free cheese squares seemed mostly made of rubber, a version of full-fat American cheese squares. The thin cellophane wrappers made them ideal for tossing into Sammi's lunch box once she went back to school, but like everything else, they returned home, sometimes crumpled under the still-full fat-free yogurt she hadn't eaten. They were so synthetic that I could smooth the whole square flat and the "cheese" wouldn't even have a crack in it.

Treats were easier to give her, made entirely of sugar and therefore naturally fat free. She got fruit snacks again and gummy bears, and my parents sent her another enormous tub of the old standard, Jelly Belly jelly beans, which had also been compatible with her last diet. What she liked most, though, sent shivers up my spine, an item I could have never predicted would show up in my house: fat-free fudge Snackwells cookies.

When I was a teenager in the 1980s, Snackwells came out with a whole line of "diet" cookies. My mother loved them, placing them on the same shelf in the kitchen on which she'd previously set the white paper bags of Pepperidge Farm cookies when my brother and I were little. There were two varieties of Snackwells that I remembered. There were the vanilla sandwich ones, which were a "special treat" for my mom—and later for my college roommate who had a full-blown eating disorder—because they were only low fat instead of fat free; and there were chocolate fudge ones, a chewy, waxy cookie without a single gram of fat. By the time I was a sophomore in high school, there were almost never any other store-bought cookies in the house, but these cookies were definitely not for me or my brother. If I begged, she'd let me have one but with the caveat that these were the only treats she could have. The implication that she was not allowed any other cookies made me feel sorry for her, but with no other cookies in the house most of the time, they still beckoned.

I had a complicated relationship with those cookies: they weren't good, but they were all we had. Eating them made me feel guilty anyway—not for the grand transgression of ingesting unneeded calories but for depriving my mother of something she was willing to allow herself, even on her diet. The many layers of agitated thinking surrounding these cookies made bile arise in my throat upon simply seeing the packaging in my roommate's pile of groceries four years later. When Sammi was required to go on a fat-free diet nearly two decades after that, I saw the logo in the grocery store during one of my first trips there and literally said aloud, "Oh shit."

If it wasn't enough to face the remnants of toxic diet culture in my pantry, I often encountered it socially when other people tried to make light of Sammi's restrictions. Half a dozen friends and family members asked me to let them know what kind of "great food discoveries" we made on this diet so that they could incorporate those foods into their weight-loss plans. When I mentioned to one family member that I couldn't wait to start feeding Sammi whole avocados and adding whipped cream to her bowls of berries, that person warned me that I'd be damning her to a life of being fat if I got her used to those flavors. Looking down at my eight-year-old's tiny body lost in a size-six button-down shirt she wore to avoid tearing her stitches out putting on a pullover, I tried to hold my tongue.

Only once, though, did I lose my temper. One morning after Sammi was able to return to school, I was waiting with her in the front office for the halls to clear so that she could walk to her classroom without fear of being jostled by the crowd. As we waited, a teacher we knew stopped us with a smile and a gentle high-five for Sammi. "How's that diet going?" she asked.

"Fine," Sammi said, looking down.

"It's rough," I admitted. "Just two and a half more weeks."

"You know what?" the teacher said, crouching down to look Sammi in the eye. "You should tell me what you're eating these days! I need to be on a diet, too. Maybe you can give me some ideas and I can be eating what you're eating!"

"No," I said sharply, pulling Sammi closer to my side. "This diet is not good for people. It's only because of what happened to Sammi in surgery, and it's only for a little while. It's not healthy to eat like this all the time. You should eat fat every day if your doctor says it's OK for you."

"Ah, who cares?" the teacher persisted with a wink. "If it gets off these winter pounds, I'm all for it! Sammi, can you make me a list of all the things you're eating?"

"No," I barked at her. "No, and that's not OK that you're suggesting it. We have to go now."

I took Sammi into the conference room at the back of the office and told her that the teacher we'd just spoken with was wrong to ask what she did. "This is a temporary diet," I said, looking her right in the eye. "I'm sorry she even tried to talk with you that way. No one should follow this diet unless their doctor says they have to!"

"I know, Momma," Sammi said, looking tired and thin. My heart was pounding, and I pulled my little daughter to my chest and stroked her thin, dry hair, more for my own good than hers. When the bell rang, I said goodbye to her and walked home, fuming.

Sammi was also, we knew, feeling the effects that eating a totally fat-free diet has on the brain's serotonin production. I knew from my own experience that low cholesterol can cause depression and anxiety; it turns out that a low (or no) fat diet has a similar effect. In Sammi, this presented as extreme agitation, amplified by the drugs she was taking to help her pass the fluid out of her chest, which messed with her electrolyte levels. She'd cry and scream that she was hungry but nothing sounded good, or she would run her hands all over her body, sobbing, telling us that she just felt "wrong." Some days she'd come home from school, sit down on the couch, and watch TV with tears streaming down her face that she couldn't explain. I'd sit next to her, hold and snuggle her, and do my best not to cry myself.

In May, just three weeks after the surgery, I sent Sammi back to Hebrew school. She'd missed her friends and teachers there, and the director had promised to call me if it seemed like the day was too long for Sammi. Walking through the grocery store in search of more fat-free provisions, I felt my phone buzz in my pocket.

"Hi there, Debi," came the voice of the religious school director. "Sammi's asking if you could please come pick her up."

I looked at my cart full of groceries, the half-unfinished list resting on top of a cantaloupe in the basket. "Of course," I answered. "Is she OK?"

"Well," the director hesitated, "I'm not sure what's going on, to tell you the truth. She was singing with her class and then, I think, her necklace fell off? She said it was a special one you'd given her, and she couldn't get it back on, and I think it just set her off."

I knew the necklace immediately. Before the surgery, I'd given Sammi and Ronni each a chain with two charms on it. I called them "good luck charms," especially chosen for each of them. Ronni's said "This is going to be the best day ever!"—a sentence she uttered so often that I'd thrilled to find it expressed in print—and "You are so loved," a reminder that she counted as much as her medically complicated little sister. Sammi's charms said "You are my sunshine," a song we sung to her so often that she'd become our "Sammi Sunshine," and "I'll eat you up I love you so," a quote from *Where the Wild Things Are*. The clasp on Sammi's chain had been doubly secure and hard for her to reattach.

"I'll be there in a few minutes," I told the director, abandoning my cart.

After I parked and walked inside the synagogue, I thought I could hear crying from the entryway. Rounding the corner and heading up the tall staircase, I was sure of it, and by the time I reached the religious school wing, I realized that the crying was Sammi. The director caught me as I began jogging toward the sound, telling me she'd gotten Ronni out of her class to keep Sammi company. The two were in the youth lounge.

I opened the door to find Ronni standing with her arms around Sammi, who was perched on a tall stool. Both looked stricken. Sammi saw me in the door of the room and howled.

"I ate fat! I ate fat! Am I going to die?"

I must have turned white, because Ronni immediately began crying, too. I raced to them and wrapped them both in my arms. Ronni explained through tears that Sammi had been upset about her necklace, so Ronni had come to talk with her while she waited for me. In Ronni's class, they were being rewarded for a good performance on a recent

Hebrew test, and they had all been given slices of pizza. Without thinking, Ronni had returned to the classroom to ask if she could get a slice for her sister, who had eaten some before they'd both realized their mistake.

"Oh, that was so nice of you," I told Ronni. I felt all the blood draining from my ankles and collapsed with them onto the nearby couch. "You just forgot! It's OK!" I told her.

But I wasn't at all sure if it was OK. I sat there holding my two traumatized children and wondered how I would ever untangle the word "fat" from the word "dangerous" for them if Sammi wasn't OK. Even if Sammi didn't need to be hospitalized, her chest full of fluid, due to this oversight, I wondered if the negative association with fat was now permanent. I held two future women, ages eleven and eight, in my arms, frozen in time, utterly terrified.

Eventually, I got out my phone to call Dr. Backer's office. I explained what had happened and asked what our next step should be.

"Just three bites, you say?" the nurse on the other end of the phone asked.

I looked at Ronni. "You're not in trouble," I told her. "I promise. But it's very important that you tell me the best you can remember about how much Sammi ate. Was it really only three bites?"

Ronni nodded seriously. "Yes. And one of the bites was really small, because it was hot," she told me.

The nurse had heard her. "That should be OK," she reassured me. "Just keep an eye on her, OK? Watch for any signs that she's having trouble breathing. Let us know, or even just come in, if you're worried."

I thanked her and got off the phone breezily. "It's OK," I told them. "Really, it will be OK. Sammi, you just have to promise to tell me if you feel icky at all, OK? Because then we'll just go get an X-ray—no ouchies—OK?"

Sammi shuddered and nodded. I picked her up under her bottom like a toddler and carried her out, sending Ronni for their backpacks and jackets. Try as I might, though, I couldn't convince Sammi to skip the school choir concert that night. She'd been so happy to have the chance to sing with her friends and didn't want to miss it, but she made me promise to stand near the stage in case she had trouble breathing or, in her words, "started to faint." I did as she asked, standing near the stage

every time she was on it, and we skittered out at the end of the evening
without saying a word to any of our concerned friends. Later that night,
I received half a dozen email messages asking what was wrong. Appar-
ently, she and I both had looked like we were at the end of our ropes.
In truth, we were.

That Friday evening, I figured out a way to make a fat-free pizza
for Sammi, desperate not to sour her on pizza forever. Using a fat-free
crust recipe, tomato sauce seasoned with basil and oregano, and fat-free
cheese, I presented her with the surprise when she came home from
school. She was excited and even jumped up and down, squealing.
There was no sign of the tear-faced little girl from Hebrew school earlier that week, and I dared to hope it had been a blip she'd remember
as a bad moment in the context of a bad diet, not the beginning of the
demonization of fat grams forever.

For Ronni, I made a regular pizza with her favorites on top. It
was not just Sammi for whom I was afraid; I was terrified that Ronni
might try to take on Sammi's diet in solidarity and then become obsessed
and unable to pull herself out. I knew being the steady, calm, reliable,
healthy older sister weighed on her even though she promised that she
felt every bit as important to us as Sammi. Every chance I got, I snuck
Ronni out for a treat or spent extra time in her room at night to listen
to her wild imaginings about Harry Potter and Hogwarts.

That night with our homemade pizzas, it was just the three of us;
David was out of town for work. We picked our movie and settled onto
the couch. In front of us on the coffee table were our pizzas and a side
of sautéed spinach, which we all usually loved. Out of the corner of my
eye, I watched Sammi nibble at her spinach and ignore her one slice of
pizza for long stretches. I paused the movie several times to ask if she
wanted me to warm it up, but she demurred. "I like it cold," she said,
as I watched the fat-free cheese congeal and reveal its rubbery texture in
the glow of the screen. On the other side of the plate, the spinach was
cold, lying limply in a puddle of the broth and crushed garlic in which
I'd cooked it.

When the movie ended, I turned the TV off and looked at Sammi.
"You barely ate anything," I told her, pointing out the obvious.

"I'm going to eat it," she said, picking up the slice of pizza and
taking a tiny bite.

"It's 7:30!" I exploded. "We sat down to eat two hours ago!"

She looked at her plate and said nothing.

"It's something you like, isn't it?" I asked her, staring over her head at the kitchen full of dishes to wash.

"Yes," she said. "But it's not fair!"

"What isn't fair?" I said, angrily piling my and Ronni's plates to take them into the kitchen. "Is it not fair that I worked hard to make this for you, and then I let you watch a movie during dinner? Is that the part that isn't fair?"

Sammi began to cry. "It's not fair that you don't know by now that I'm a slow eater!" she said, tears running down her face.

"Oh, I *know* you're a slow eater. I do know that. I know it very, very well, kid," I said, walking away from her into the kitchen.

Underneath my unleashed resentment, I was aware that I was an adult losing my temper with a child only a month out from major cardiac surgery, a child with more than eight years of horribly twisted anatomy in her immediate muscle memory. I knew, even as I said what I was about to say, that I would regret it. I knew that I'd been pushed too far; that if David had been home, I wouldn't have said it; that I would need to forgive myself later—but I was over the edge now after years of standing at the stove and walking through the grocery store in service of the caloric needs of this little girl who refused to eat the pizza I'd made her. I was done.

"Maybe," I said, walking back to the living room where Sammi still clutched her pizza, "we should just ask the doctor to put in a feeding tube."

"No!" she cried.

"I'm serious," I told her, though I wasn't. "Maybe it would be better for you and I not to constantly fight about food. Maybe if you got all your food through a tube down your throat, we could talk about something else sometimes, and you wouldn't have to worry about how fast you ate, and I wouldn't have to worry about doctors telling me that I don't feed you enough."

Sammi cried, the pizza held in the air. "You do feed me enough!" she said.

"Well, obviously not," I said. "Obviously, what I make isn't good enough. I give up."

With that, I left her sitting at the table in the living room and went to the kitchen to do dishes. Ronni hovered between the two rooms, not sure what to do.

"I'm frustrated," I told her as I scrubbed the pot where the pizza sauce had cooked. "It's not anyone's fault, but I'm not good company right now. Would you go keep your sister company while she finishes?"

Ronni nodded then stopped. "She's just still slow, Momma," she told me.

I finished the dishes while Ronni talked with Sammi. *Would it never be over?* I wondered. Years of cooking for special diets, months of waiting for the surgery that would help, and now, after it all, we were no better off. At bedtime, I told Sammi I was sorry I'd lost my temper.

"I'm sorry I didn't eat my pizza during the movie," she said.

When I came downstairs, I went outside, sat on the back steps, and cried.

Still, through all of it, I persevered. Knowing there was a deadline for this wretched diet was helpful, and we all but marked it off in X's on the wall. After the pizza debacle, I vowed to find one meal that we all enjoyed and that could be customized to accommodate everyone and to institute a new tradition that became the cornerstone of the six-week diet and beyond. We called it "Sushi Movie Shabbos."

The previous summer, my friend Rebecca had taught us to make sushi rolls. Because I have a serious fish allergy, I'd tried sushi only once, in a vegan restaurant where I knew cross-contamination with fish wasn't possible, but after our friends showed us how to make rolls at home, we'd gotten creative with it. Sitting on the couch one day with Sammi after school, I thought about the ingredients involved. Like a Rolodex with cards sliding out into the air in front of me, I ticked them off one by one.

Vegetables: We had to omit avocado, but tomatoes, cucumbers, bell peppers, carrots, and scallions were all fat free.

Rice: I searched the web and found that short-grain rice was entirely fat free.

Tamagoyaki: The special sweetened, layered omelet we often made to stuff our rolls would be just as easy to make with egg whites, I realized. By then, I'd started buying egg whites in quart-sized cartons.

Seaweed: This one worried me—wasn't it cooked in oil? But it turned out to be a negligible amount. Seaweed was OK.

Soy sauce: Fat free!

Pickled ginger: Fat free!

And, as if in answer to the question I'd been asking myself, Susan texted me from the grocery store that day with a photo, which she'd been doing for the last few weeks whenever she saw something fat free she thought I might find interesting. That day, miraculously, it was fat-free cream cheese, the ingredient that would round out our sushi rolls.

The next Friday, I declared our Shabbos (Yiddish for "sabbath") meal to be sushi, which we would eat in the living room in front of the TV, something we'd seldom done before due to exactly what had happened the week before with the pizza. Engaged in conversation and holding a bite of food on a fork for minutes at a time, Sammi still forgot to eat even at the dining room table; watching TV made it harder for David and me to keep track of what she ate and remind her to continue eating. However, we needed something to prevent us from losing patience while sitting at the dining room table for hours every night waiting for Sammi to finish. All four of us really needed, for the sake of our relationship, to look away from each other for a few hours. This new tradition of forced reprieve from worry seemed like the only way to move forward.

Every Friday night for the remainder of the chylothorax diet—even during the two low-fat weeks that followed the fat-free ones—I made four plates of sushi rolls: one with fat-free cream cheese for Sammi; one with fat-free ingredients that we could all eat; one with full-fat dairy and avocado for David and Ronni; and one with vegan cream cheese for me. The meal, with all its color and symmetry and elegance, came to represent a movement toward serenity in our eating habits and our attitudes. We each took on specific tasks involved in the creation of our Sushi Movie Shabbos nights that endured long past the chylothorax diet or even Sammi's challenges regarding eating in general. I always prepared the eggs and started the rice cooker; Ronni always sliced the grape tomatoes; Sammi and I rolled the sushi; and David took his station at the counter near the stove to slice the rolls perfectly and set them out on the trays. Seamlessly, the table was set with the navy and white melamine plates and the shallow, pale blue ramekins in which we poured soy sauce and David and I squeezed thick green wasabi paste. In front of *The King and I*, *The Little Princess*, *My Neighbor Totoro*, and several other movies I've since forgotten, I watched Sammi only occasionally, out of the corner of one eye, as she precariously balanced a piece of sushi in her "cheater" chopsticks, holding it in midair.

For dessert, the rice in our bellies continuing to expand and fill us, we ate big bowls of deep red strawberries. For an hour or two, full of vinegary rice and the sharp tang of red peppers, we were content, suspended in the place between surgery and the new Sammi.

10

SUMMER LUNCH BOX

After six weeks of the fat-free diet, I took Sammi to the children's hospital for an X-ray. If they saw no "pleural effusion"—in other words, leaking chyle or other fluids around her lungs—then she would graduate to the next step in her recovery: a low-fat diet. We took our usual path through the hospital parking lot, across a sun-drenched stretch of carpeted hallway, to the interior elevators down to radiology.

In the radiology room, Sammi dutifully lifted off her shirt, stretched her arms around the X-ray panel, and displayed her pink, healing incision to the room. I noted the prominence of her ribs, the dryness of her skin, the resignation of her posture. If I didn't think too hard about it, most of the time I could forget that most other children didn't know the rhythms and requirements of hospital visits like this; that most other children wouldn't know how to stand for a chest X-ray, how to wait with a gas mask over their faces for surgery, or even think to ask their mothers whether this visit would be to go to sleep or stay awake. But sometimes, like when I saw her simply grab the sidebars around the X-ray machine as she had so many other times, it hit me that she was now a semiprofessional hospital patient. Exhaustion settled over me in those moments like a weighted blanket. *What had we done to her?*

Unlike the wait for endoscopy results, though, the wait for X-ray results was very short.

"It looks great, Mom," the radiology technician called out. "No fluid. She can move on to the low-fat diet."

"Yay!" Sammi called out from the doorway of the room where she'd put her clothes back on. "Mommy, do you have the Junior Mints?"

The day before, we'd had brunch with David's family, and his sister Sherri had asked Sammi what she wanted to eat first if she was able to begin the low-fat diet today. Sammi had grinned from ear to ear.

"*Seven* Junior Mints!" she answered, nearly bouncing out of her chair.

"Why seven?" Sherri had pressed her. "Is seven your favorite number?"

"Because until now," I'd explained, "she could have only three Junior Mints at a time."

Everyone at the table had been quiet for a moment then. I'd been horrified by the idea of doling out three at a time, too—it seemed like the kind of cruel restriction I'd heard about from gymnastics coaches or ballet dancers—but Sammi simply had been happy to have any "real" chocolate. The idea had come from the pamphlets we got from the hospital, but when I did the math, the low-fat diet allowed for about three times the number of Junior Mints per serving. Just to be careful, though, and to leave room for other sources of fat in her snacks, I'd decided on seven. I knew that our extended family had believed us when we told them how hard this diet had been, but moments like that—seeing how they registered and then quickly covered their shock—I could see the realization spread across their faces. Some of them looked at their laps and others plastered big smiles on their faces, doing their best to be excited about the seven mints, right along with Sammi. Though I had been living it for weeks by then, seeing them grasp the truly obsessive level of fat-gram counting required by this diet brought tears to my eyes. I wiped them away as I walked to the kitchen for a bowl of strawberries.

Heading back to the car after the X-ray the following week, I handed Sammi the bag of candy. She opened it and pulled out one mint, nibbling a bite from it and smiling. From half a gram of fat per meal, we had now graduated to one-and-a-half grams. I thought it would be a revelation, but it was not. When we got home, I made Sammi a half-serving bowl of air-popped popcorn (1 gram of fat) and half of a low-fat string cheese (0.5 grams of fat). As I prepared that night's dinner in the kitchen, I peeked in on her where she sat with her snacks in the living room while watching TV. Sammi barely touched them, just holding a piece of popcorn to her lips without moving.

When Ronni came home from middle school, she smelled the popcorn and shouted with glee. "Can I have some, Sammi?" she asked. By the time I checked again, Ronni was holding the bowl in her lap, and almost all the popcorn was gone. When I went back to the living room half an hour later, the girls were settling into their homework at our kitchen counter, and the string cheese still sat limply on the coffee table.

The week of low-fat food passed largely in the same way the six weeks preceding it had; I cooked food only mildly more flavorful than what we'd eaten before, and Sammi ate it with performed enthusiasm but actual apathy. She dragged herself through breakfast, brought home her low-fat lunch mostly uneaten, and picked at dinner. I held my breath as I listened to hers, carefully, asking casually about whether she felt any different.

"Breathing OK?" I probed, my back to her.

"Yep," came the answer as she hoisted herself onto the stool.

On May 29, the last day of the low-fat diet, I took her out of school for the whole day. If she had made it through this diet with no chyle leaking through her chest, I resolved that we would go out for an amazing meal and visit the nearest chocolate shop. If not, we would go to the nearby American Girl store and distract her with some new doll clothes while I figured out what was next. It was impossible to imagine her X-ray showing any chyle leak though; she seemed fine.

I was right. Her X-ray showed a normal chest cavity, and what's more, Dr. Backer's advanced practice nurse surprised us by telling us that this would be our last visit with them. Just seven weeks after the surgery to sew her aorta to her chest wall, Sammi was released from the care of the cardiothoracic surgeon for good.

We stepped out into the busy streets of downtown Chicago and stared up at a deep blue sky. "You are in charge of lunch," I told Sammi. "If you tell me what you want, I will get us there, absolutely anywhere or anything you want. But first I have a surprise for you."

I led her across busy Michigan Avenue and past the historic water tower into the Hershey Store. As we walked inside, I squeezed her hand. "Pick out whatever you want," I told her. "You've been so good about taking care of your body this whole time. It was hard, and you did it anyway. Go nuts, kiddo. *Anything* you want!"

She squealed in delight. I tried to put myself in her place—denied treats for eight weeks, what would I want first? I let my eyes drift over super-sized Hershey Kisses, enormous bags of Reese's Peanut Butter Cups, and tubes of Rolo caramels. If not for my own lactose intolerance, I would have gone nuts right alongside her. I watched as she wandered from item to item, trying to choose.

"Momma!" she called. "Look!"

Anxious to see what her first choice was, I rounded a display and found her holding a giant pillow shaped like a unicorn. "It smells like cotton candy!" she cooed. "Here, smell it!"

Dutifully, I smelled it. "But you can't eat that," I teased. "Come on, pick something you can eat!"

"OK, Momma," she answered, putting down the pillow. "But could I have a pillow instead of candy?"

"No," I said, "not today. Today is the day for treats! You're not so excited about treats?"

"No, I'm excited," she said quickly. "I am."

Just then, a store employee approached us. "Would you like a Hershey's Kiss?" she offered sweetly, "if your mom says it's OK."

"It's totally OK," I answered. "Go ahead, Sunshine."

Sammi stood against a backdrop of candy and carefully unwrapped her Kiss. I pulled out my phone and snapped a photo just as she was about to bite into it. I marveled at the ways in which she seemed different from me in that moment. If I hadn't had real chocolate in eight weeks, I would have gobbled that Kiss. She took a nibble off the top, gave me an exaggerated swoon, and carried it around the store, taking little bites from it for the next several minutes. By the time she finished it, there was melted chocolate on her hands.

We finally left the store with a bag of miniature York Peppermint Patties and a bag of York-flavored candy-coated chocolates. "Let's have dessert first," I insisted, and we sat on the sidewalk against the wall of the store. I pulled out a piece of vegan chocolate I'd brought for myself and took a bite.

As I chewed, I watched Sammi unwrap her chocolates carefully and then take bites out of treats that were labeled "bite sized." In the bright May sun, her skin looked translucent—pale with pink cheeks, tiny burst blood vessels near the corners of her eyes and lips—and her hair showed every frayed end as she tucked it behind her ears. She'd worn a dress for our big day in the city, and it hung loosely on her. For my own sake, I'd stopped monitoring her weight, but it was obvious that she was thinner than before the surgery. Though I'd been imagining this adventure as a bacchanal of fatty foods, I'd failed to admit to myself what I knew: Sammi couldn't overeat. She didn't even know how to eat *enough*. After two miniature York patties and a few candy-coated chocolate pieces, she looked up at me and said, "I'm done for now. Could you put these in your purse?"

Once again, I struggled with my disappointment. My agenda for the day—eating and regaining ground—quickly felt futile. I put the chocolate in my purse and asked, though I knew what she'd say, if she wanted to go out for lunch now.

"No," she said predictably. "I'm full from the candy."

Instead, we went to the Lego store, spending forty-five minutes creating hilarious figurine mashups of Harry Potter and Batman, animals, and people. Then we went to American Girl Place and looked at every new outfit available for her doll, McKenna, and her sister's doll, and her friends' dolls, and all the accessories. As we walked from one robust young girl doll to another, I felt my inner monitor of Sammi's daily food intake begin to sound an alarm. It was early afternoon now, and she hadn't asked for lunch.

Eventually, I put my hands on her shoulders as she gazed lovingly at the newest doll. "It's two o'clock," I said, "and I think maybe we should get lunch."

We walked to the upscale food court in the basement where Sammi agreed to a slice of pizza and some french fries. Again, I took a photo of her in front of her food, a french fry held delicately between her teeth. During the hour we sat there, I finished my lunch, and she talked about American Girl dolls between small nibbles of her fries and pizza. When an hour had passed, I asked if she was done.

She was.

We wrapped the pizza in foil. On our way back to the car, a department store employee standing in front of a branded truck was handing out free sunglasses, and Sammi gleefully chose zebra-striped ones. We took our last photo of the day, a selfie, sundrenched and backlit, our sunglasses obscuring the worry in my eyes.

A few weeks later—nearly three months after the surgery that un-kinked Sammi's esophagus—she was still not eating well. I took her to see Dr. Lynn, her pediatrician, for a follow-up appointment.

"She had a swallow study before we left the hospital," I said, my hand on Sammi's knee. "Everything is moving through her esophagus perfectly now."

"That's great," Dr. Lynn smiled. "So you can eat just fine now, huh?"

Sammi nodded.

"Does it feel different?" she asked her. "Like, is it easier?"

"Yeah!" Sammi said. "Water is so cold when it gets to my stomach!"

"What about food, though?" Dr. Lynn pressed her. "Does the food go down faster now?"

"Kinda," Sammi answered, looking at me.

"Mom?" Dr. Lynn turned to me. "Why's she looking at you for the answer?"

I explained that Sammi was still eating very slowly and that I was worried that she didn't quite trust that it wasn't going to come back up in her mouth anymore.

"It's not going to come back up, Sammi," Dr. Lynn said, her back turned as she washed her hands. "It's all better in there. You can take big bites now, OK? And tell mom I said you can eat some junk food if you want it."

"OK," Sammi answered.

"Now let's take a look at that incision. Can you pull off that shirt for me?"

Sammi pulled off her T-shirt. Dr. Lynn ran a finger over the scar that had formed and told us she was impressed with Dr. Backer's work. It wasn't raised or bumpy; it had healed beautifully.

When Sammi left to go to the bathroom, I asked Dr. Lynn about something I remembered from when Sammi was a baby: feeding ther-apy. Before Sammi's ear tubes were put in, the ENT who'd discovered her double aortic arch had sent us for a few sessions of feeding therapy to assess whether Sammi *could* swallow foods. We'd been dismissed once we knew what the problem really was, but I wondered if that was some-thing to revisit now.

In Dr. Lynn's office nearly eight years later, I asked about it. "Should she be seeing someone to, I don't know, kind of *relearn* how to eat properly?"

"Nah," Dr. Lynn answered as she stood up from where she was taking notes on her chart. "She just needs some time. Remember, Mom, she's been eating like that her whole life. It's going to take her some time to trust that she isn't going to gag. Just be patient."

I tried, but I wasn't optimistic. Right on cue, just a few days later, Sammi came home from school with a completely full lunch box. I knew that she hadn't eaten more than half a bowl of cereal for breakfast, so I asked her what she'd eaten at school that day.

"I couldn't eat at lunch!" she sobbed suddenly. "My friend Bryce was mean to me and I felt too sad to eat!"

"OK," I answered, wrapping my arms around her. "OK, I get it. Does anything sound good right now? You must be so hungry!"

"Could I have popcorn?" she sniffled.

I acquiesced, desperate for her to eat something. By dinnertime, she'd eaten a bowl or two of popcorn and had no appetite for the beans and rice she'd requested earlier.

After she went to bed, I mused about calling Dr. Lynn again to ask for help. In the file folders of my mind, I skimmed over snippets of conversations online, comments made in passing by doctors or nurses, things I'd read, things I'd wondered. I scrubbed the pots of beans and rice and tried to remember the name of the appetite-stimulating drug someone had mentioned in the early days of her reflux.

Was it periactin? Should I ask for that? What will Dr. Lynn think if I ask for a drug by name? Am I one of those *parents? I read it on a message board and now I think I know better than the doctor. She said to wait. . . . She said to be patient. . . .*

I set the pot on the stove to dry and turned to the cutting boards. *Maybe she can't chew correctly. They had us stimulate her gums when she was in feeding therapy as a baby. . . . Did we give up on that too fast? Maybe we should have seen them again after the surgery. Should I have pushed for therapy all along?*

Therapy. Oh my G-d, she's got such a messed-up relationship with food. She's going to end up starving when she goes to college. She'll never eat without someone there to tell her. Does she have an eating disorder? Did we do that to her with all these diets? We made food dangerous. Citrus, chocolate, tomatoes, dairy, soy, eggs, nuts, wheat, fat—what's left?

She can't live on popcorn and raspberries. How are we going to fix this? How?

"Mommy?" Sammi's voice jolted me out of my thoughts. I turned away from the sink to see her standing at the entrance to the kitchen, tear-stained, shuddering, holding her doll, and staring at me with pleading eyes.

I put down the measuring cups I was washing and dried my hands on my jeans. "Oh sweetie, what's going on?" I asked, picking her up and walking toward the couch.

"I . . . want to sleep . . . but . . . I can't sleep!" she sobbed.

"Well, that happens sometimes," I said. "There's even a name for it."

"There is?"

"Yes," I said, smoothing her hair away from her face. "It's called *insomnia.*"

"Oh."

"Why do you think you can't sleep?" I asked, settling her against my chest.

Sammi started crying again, harder this time. "I don't know!" she howled.

She cried like that, lying in my lap on the couch in the darkened living room, for several minutes. I tried the trick I'd employed when she was a baby. I made my breathing deeper and slower, counting in my head to keep the beats even. It had calmed her when she was tiny. It worked, a little, all these years later. She breathed haltingly but stopped crying, then eventually pulled her arm out from around me to rest her hand against my cheek.

"It's OK to be awake," I said finally. "You don't have to sleep to rest your body."

I reminded her that there is value in lying quietly in bed, appreciating the comfort of the blankets, the smells of home, and the sounds of the people in the house. "Keeping your body still is not as restful as sleeping, but it's good for us," I told Sammi. "And knowing that makes me not so worried about not sleeping when insomnia happens to me."

She was quiet again and then, in a small voice, asked if I would stay with her until she fell asleep.

"Sure," I said.

I left the rest of the dishes to soak, put on my own pajamas, and took my laptop up to the hallway outside Sammi's room. I tucked her back into bed and then sat in the doorframe.

Talking to Sammi about insomnia reminded me of my awful bouts with it during the first year of her life. I thought about all the late-night online Messenger conversations I'd had with Hilary that year. Both of us were struggling with postpartum mood issues then, but with Sammi about three months older than Hilary's child, I'd been going through it a little longer. As we sent messages to each other during my late nights and her midmornings, I'd remind her of something my midwife had told me when Ronni was a baby.

"A woman can go without good sleep or good food," I'd typed, "but not both. Make sure you're eating."

Of course, I also knew that I wasn't as capable of following that advice as I was at doling it out. Being anxious and tired sapped my appetite, and I hadn't been much of a cook then. I'd survived on those Starbucks hot chocolates and either toast or cookies most of the time. In retrospect, some of my insomnia might very well have been my body's refusal to rest until it was properly nourished, though I didn't know it then.

Thinking about this outside Sammi's bedroom, I flashed on another memory. When David's grandmother was alive, she had told me that she could never sleep if she was hungry. "I have to have something before I go to bed," she said. "Even just a glass of milk." Sammi, I suddenly realized, might not be able to sleep because—of course—she was *hungry*. Her bedroom was above mine and David's, and for years we'd heard her shuffle around her room, climb up and down the ladder to her loft bed, and turn on the comedy albums she listened to several times at night before finally falling asleep. Despite all I'd done to feed her—for years now—she was badly malnourished. This would not get better with waiting; the clarity I needed had interrupted my reverie at the sink for a reason.

I needed more than a medication for her, I realized. I wanted to solve the root of the problem. I felt sure it was no longer outside her control—seeing the marshmallow fluff go down smoothly during her last swallow study was proof. If her challenge was chewing, conditioned emotional reactions to foods, or simply muscle memory, the right solution was feeding therapy. I searched "feeding issues children heart esophagus," and the answer was on the first page I opened.

The website of the American Speech-Language-Hearing Association listed potential causes of feeding and swallowing disorders in children:

- reflux or other stomach problems
- being premature or having a low birth weight
- heart disease
- sensory issues
- behavior problems

Searching further, I found the website for Stanford University's children's hospital, which added more potential causes, including:

- large tonsils
- irritation or scarring of the esophagus or vocal cords by acid in gastroesophageal reflux disease (GERD)
- compression of the esophagus by other body parts, such as enlargements of the heart, thyroid gland, blood vessels, or lymph nodes

I checked these items off in my head, one after the other. Sammi had experienced every single one of them.

The next morning, I called the nearest feeding therapy practice I could find. A half hour's drive away, I thought it would be worth every mile and every penny if they could help teach Sammi to eat. I didn't call Dr. Lynn; though I appreciated her candor and her refusal to join me in my panic, I needed someone to take my worry seriously this time. It was simply too hard to continue this way, waiting for Sammi to believe in her own body's ability to swallow without discomfort.

The pediatric feeding therapy practice was in the basement of a nondescript office building. The first day we went, I brought both girls, explaining to them that we were there to meet with someone who might be able to help Sammi trust in her healthy esophagus and eat a little faster so she could grow. Ronni, by then twelve years old, waited in the lobby while Sammi and I met with the therapist. Just like the feeding therapists had when Sammi was a baby, this practice asked us to bring her feeling hungry. We arrived at 8:30 a.m. with a lunch box containing a covered bowl of cereal and a container of soy milk as well as small container of raspberries. By then, Sammi had been awake for more than two hours.

"It's so nice to meet you, Sammi," said Margot, the feeding therapist. She wore a bright green dress with a Peter Pan collar, and her big smile and blue eyes won over Sammi from the very first moment. She led us to an office with a small, plastic picnic table in it, and motioned for us to sit down across from her.

First, Margot asked both Sammi and me to articulate our goals. I explained, as briefly as I could, the history of Sammi's challenges with eating. I told her about the initial surgery and the first short stint of feeding therapy; what I had started to label as her misdiagnosis with eosinophilic esophagitis; and the recent surgery to free her esophagus, including the recovery with the fat-free diet. I said I wanted Sammi to be able to eat easily, without pain or emotional upset, and I wanted our family to be able to finish a meal in less than an hour.

"That seems like a very reasonable goal, Mom," Margot answered, turning to Sammi. "What about you, Sammi? What do you want to accomplish?"

Sammi shrugged, though her mouth betrayed the hint of a nervously excited smile.

"Is there anything *you* want to make sure we work on together?" Margot pressed her.

"Eat faster so I can play?" Sammi said, squirming.

"I love that idea!" Margot answered. "I'm going to write that down: *more time for playing.* OK, Mom," she continued, turning to me. "I think Sammi and I can take it from here. You can go wait in the waiting room, and we'll come get you when we're ready to share what we've worked on."

"OK," I smiled, standing up. "Sammi, you saw where the waiting room is. If you need me, just come get me, OK?"

"OK," Sammi answered, already turning toward Margot.

Just like that, I was closing the door behind me and walking back toward the waiting room. I hadn't even brought a book; I'd thought I would be in the appointment with Sammi this time. For the next thirty minutes, I stared at my phone in silence as Ronni read next to me.

For the sessions that followed, I always brought a book; I was seldom even invited into the room. For the first time, Sammi was addressing her health without me there. Going forward, the sessions took place during lunch, and Sammi would bring her school lunch box packed with the things she chose: quesadillas, of course, but also potato chips, the ubiquitous containers of fruit, Oreos, and chopped avocado, all accompanied by the cup of Carnation Instant Breakfast. I sat in the waiting room and read, curious, as Margot and Sammi ate together and made plans. Every week, they emerged with Sammi grinning ear to ear, a half-sheet of blue paper in her hand. She'd hand it to me, and I would read a list of assignments for each of us, with variations:

SAMMI'S ASSIGNMENTS:
  1. *Finish half of my Carnation Instant Breakfast by 1:00 p.m.*
  2. *Take bites of dinner while I listen to my family talk*
  3. *Have a bedtime snack*

MOMMY'S ASSIGNMENTS:
  1. *Don't say "please finish" or "take another bite"*
  2. *Give me Cheez-Its to take to camp*
  3. *Give me a bedtime snack even if I don't finish dinner*

Margot would explain the rationale for the assignments, and Sammi would smile and show me her lunch box with half a quesadilla gone, absent most of the raspberries, and a notable volume of Carnation Instant Breakfast missing from the cup. "Look how much I ate!" she'd gloat.

"I bet your tummy feels full!" I'd answer, matching her enthusiasm.

At home, the work continued. Sammi reminded me gently when I said, "Hey, sweetie, you do need to finish lunch before we go to camp," that *not* telling her to finish was on my list of goals. I held my tongue as much as I could. When the bottle of Carnation Instant Breakfast languished, full, on the kitchen counter, I wordlessly took it to her where she sat on the couch. Every week, we returned to the therapy practice for another mystery appointment. Every week, I was reminded not to nag her.

I sat in the windowless waiting room on an orange plastic chair, staring at the industrial carpeting between my feet every week that summer, anxiously clenching my jaw. Though even the gastroenterologist had told me that I could not make Sammi grow just by feeding her more calories, I'd spent her entire life trying to feed her. Stepping back from that role left me feeling powerless. Besides, I was not convinced that the entire experience wasn't an enormous waste of time. Though Sammi loved the control she suddenly had over my and David's behavior at mealtimes—and even more so, the unquestioned access to "bedtime snacks"—I didn't see evidence that she was gaining weight or eating more quickly. Too, we'd begun, at an achingly slow pace, to wean Sammi off of her PPI medication, again, and I felt taut and watchful, alert for the signs that she was gagging or retching.

Regardless, we returned week after week to this place that I simultaneously hoped would teach her to eat while also hoping that it was entirely unnecessary. After all, if she could learn to eat here, then I'd failed to teach her myself. If she couldn't learn here, with professionals, then we were doomed, but at least it wasn't my fault. I wrestled with these conflicting feelings as I stared at the floor then painted a smile on my face the minute Sammi and Margot came through the door.

"Nice lunch?" I'd ask cheerily, hand in hand with Sammi as we climbed the stairs toward the parking lot.

"Yeah!" Sammi would answer simply, swinging her lunch box in her free hand.

Toward the end of June, a friend of ours offered to host a celebratory ice-cream-sundae-making competition in honor of Sammi's recovery. Having been diagnosed with juvenile diabetes as a child, he remembered the feeling of not being allowed to eat whatever he wanted. In our backyard, he loaded the table with a variety of ice creams and toppings and then announced that bragging rights would go to the person who concocted the most outrageous, decadent, glorious sundae of the group.

The adults and children lined up at the table, hooting and laughing over what we might add to our bowls. The kids jostled each other, filling their bowls and then posing with wide eyes for the obligatory photos I took of each sundae. From Ronni and our friends' children, the photos boasted huge exaggerated grins, a collection of bug-eyed, I-can't-believe-it delight at the level of indulgence they were permitted.

They'd filled their bowls to the top with ice cream, whipped cream, chocolate and caramel sauces, mini marshmallows and chocolate chips, mini Oreo cookies, and maraschino cherries. They were giddy.

For Sammi, though, the photo betrayed the battle she was still facing. She was drowning in her clothes, a tiny green T-shirt and flowing summer pants hiding her thin frame even under the too-big pink fleece jacket that Ronni had outgrown at age seven. Sammi was smiling, but her eyes were unfocused. It was almost as if she knew that this was supposed to be fun, but she didn't understand why.

A little while later, I walked over to where she sat on the ground with her friends. "Hey, your ice cream will melt if you leave it too long," I told her, pointing at the bowl next to her on the picnic blanket.

"It's OK," she said, craning her neck to look at me. "I only got a little ice cream and a *lot* of marshmallows. See?" She poked her spoon into the bowl, unearthing a mound of marshmallows from under the chocolate sauce she'd poured on top. Sure enough, there was a sliver of vanilla ice cream on the bottom, but the rest was marshmallows.

I made myself grin. "That's one way to do it!" I said with what I hoped was believable cheer. When I made my way back to the group of adults sitting around the table, I tried not to keep looking, but I couldn't help myself. Every time I checked, the bowl was on the blanket.

When will this kid finally eat? I wondered.

11

PICKLES IN LIMBO

That whole summer after Sammi's surgery felt like I was standing on the threshold between two worlds: one in which my whole life revolved around Sammi's health, the other an amorphous space made up of whatever other parents used to fill their time with their children. I balanced on the thin strip dividing these worlds, teetering on the balls of my feet, one day leaning hard into the past, another peering into the future with secretive, tentative hope.

We had spent nearly nine years hearing that Sammi would feel better and be able to eat well if only we did what the doctors had told us: teach her to sleep on her own; give her a specific medication; have tubes put in her ears; repair her vascular ring; feed her a special diet; give her even more medication. None of those things had solved the problem, and though I trusted Dr. Backer and his team this time more than I ever had before, I still couldn't see enough improvement in Sammi's eating habits to be sure this last bit of medical trauma wasn't just another empty promise. Years of scolding her about her eating only to find out later that she truly hadn't been capable of it made me loathe to push her now, and anyway, "don't nag Sammi to eat another bite" was on my assignment sheet from the feeding therapist.

Just as I had in the summer after the six-food elimination diet, I turned to cookbooks and recipe blogs to busy my worried hands. We were free—really and truly free—and I was going to enjoy it. If the summer of 2010 had been all about cookies and cupcakes, the summer of 2014 was dedicated to cakes and pies. Since I was forbidden to overtly nag Sammi about her eating, I decided to combine my curiosity about pastry with my stealthy habit of hiding calories in her favorite foods. We'd long graduated from the blueberries-and-coconut-oil trick, but I wondered how I might make desserts that tempted her more than the ice cream sundaes had. The trick, I decided, was fruit.

Ronni, at age twelve, had become one of my best sous chefs. By then I understood the chemistry of baking and the way flavors combined, but Ronni understood decorating. Side by side, we experimented with frosting piping tips and food coloring, purchasing tools we agreed we absolutely needed from the shelves of the local craft store's baking aisle. When we discovered the offset spatula—a backward-bent flexible blade perfect for smoothing the frosting on the outside of a layer cake—we knew we were ready to attempt three-tier cakes.

It was the Fourth of July when, for absolutely no reason, we decided on a lemon blueberry layer cake.

Only once we'd begun did we think to decorate it for the holiday, digging through the fridge for the green cardboard tubs of raspberries and strawberries. It was the third wonderful year we'd had a midweek farmers market in the little park just three blocks from our house. We'd amble over in the afternoons to find a handful of friends there, too, shopping for fruit from a Michigan farm that drove there every week with a truck full of treasure. Sometimes, I'd buy a tub of berries and plop down into the grass with a friend, sending Sammi and Ronni off with a tub of their own to share with their friends on the playground. We'd need to buy another round to take home. It was paradise, sitting in the sun-warmed grass, the sound of all the children playing, friends phasing in and out of the loose circles we made wherever we happened to be when we encountered each other. When the mosquitoes came out at dusk, whoever was left would stand, smacking at their calves, and call to their kids that it was time to go. There was a lazy communal joy tickling my feet in the grass. Every berry we ate during the rest of the week made me smile.

On the Fourth of July, Ronni and I baked our lemon cake studded with fresh blueberries from the farm and began making the vanilla frosting as Sammi sat at the counter, meticulously licking the lemony batter off of the beaters. I mixed the shortening, vegan butter, and powdered sugar in the giant stand mixer my mother-in-law had given me as a gift during the six-food elimination diet, adding vanilla and lemon extracts. Nearby, Ronni thinly sliced strawberries and chose the most perfect-looking slivers to adorn the top of the cake. Every so often,

Sammi would slide off her stool to reach up and snag a blueberry from the carton next to Ronni, and Ronni humored her tiny giggle as she snuck away.

"Hey, I'm missing a blueberry!" she'd call. "Has anybody seen my blueberry? About this big, kind of dark purple?" From her seat at the counter, Sammi would giggle again.

This moment, I realized as we slid one layer of the cake onto the heavy glass cake stand, was exactly what I'd always wanted. I was baking with my daughters. We were smudged with flour and powdered sugar; the counter was a mess of sticky strawberry juice and smears of frosting; and we were happily singing along to the soundtrack from the musical *Wicked*, to which we'd taken Ronni a few months prior. When I stepped back after frosting all three layers completely, Ronni stood on her tiptoes to get a good look at the top before carefully arranging slices of strawberries and whole blueberries across the top and sides. As she deliberated, I lifted Sammi off her stool to swing her around while Ronni hit all the high notes in "Defying Gravity."

This, I thought, *is how a kitchen should feel.* I loved the mess, the laughter, the creating and tasting and the pride that came with the final product, sitting triumphantly on a clean counter after the work was done. Without the mental gymnastics required by a restrictive diet, my constantly calculating brain could focus on everything else: flavor, texture, design, and—most importantly—enjoyment. That lemon-blueberry cake was our first-ever successful layer cake, and I appreciated everything about the process of making it, the delight I felt seeing the perfect layers in the first slice on my plate, and how much fun it had been to make it with Ronni.

Next, we tried a fruit tart, pressing a shortbread crust into a fluted tart pan. We baked it and then layered on a homemade custard made with soaked cashews and almond extract, exuding a perfumed scent that made me want to eat it all up with a spoon. With strawberries, raspberries, and blueberries, we built an intricate, carefully spaced spiral across the top. For the final step, Sammi stood on a stool at the counter and painted glaze onto each berry with a brand-new paintbrush. When Susan came over for brunch the next day, she oohed and aahed, praising the kids for their fancy dessert. I stood back, pleased, and reveled in having made something not just "pretty good given the dietary restrictions," but very good, period.

All summer, Sammi and I made the drive back and forth to her feeding therapy appointments once a week. I continued to wrestle with my unsettled feelings, commanded to keep to myself any comments that betrayed the worry I was feeling. I tried to hide the vigilance, training myself to care less, to let Sammi be the master of her own hunger and cravings, to let her learn on her own that food was no longer her enemy. Some days, I was more successful than others. Whenever I felt the urge to nag her clawing its way up my chest, I pulled out another recipe book.

I'd come a long way from the canned-vegetables-and-couscous cuisine of my pre-married life. By the summer after Sammi's big surgery, we were in our seventh year of subscribing to a local farm's CSA program. Every week, we walked through a beautifully landscaped yard to the garage where the farm boxes were stored for pickup. Inside, we blinked in the darkness until our eyes adjusted, then peeled open the waxed cardboard boxes to reveal the abundance of organic produce that awaited us. In a mostly empty box in the middle of the room were all the items that subscribers didn't want, and we traded, discarded, and supplemented our own box's contents all summer, swapping cilantro (which I hated so much that I couldn't even bring it inside my house) for extra arugula; pea shoots for cucumbers; giant daikon radishes for beets that, when we cut them open, were swirled pink and white like candy. Transferring the contents of our box to our own canvas sacks, we drove home with the car smelling like living soil, aromatic herbs, and sunshine.

The first summer that we'd subscribed to the CSA, they'd sent us a cookbook that took us through the growing season, vegetable by vegetable, and so I experimented, fussed, chopped, and preserved as much as I could to last us through the winter. Already I knew how to pulverize and freeze flattened bags full of all kinds of cooking greens, and the summer after Sammi's surgery, I tackled kohlrabi (made into hash browns), finally demystified garlic shoots (minced and cooked with greens), and turned every kind of summer squash we got into its own version of zucchini bread. By summer's end, my freezer was stocked with preserved vegetables and at least half a dozen loaves of zucchini/squash bread.

Despite her inability to eat enough, Sammi actually had a very adventurous palate. She would try anything and was quick to tell me she liked it, even if that didn't mean she'd gobble it up quickly. She nibbled enthusiastically at the zucchini bread when it was warm from the oven but ignored it afterward. She gave me an animated, choreographed series of both thumbs up for my first batch of shakshuka, an Israeli dish made of eggs poached in a thick tomato and garlic stew—but only finished about half an egg. When I made cashew-based pesto using the small bunch of fresh basil that had come in that week's farm box, she said it smelled "so yummy" but then left a third of it in her bowl. It wasn't what I was cooking that was the problem; it was something she'd have to work out on her own.

With the end of summer—and her approaching dismissal from feeding therapy for "good progress" that seemed negligible to me—Sammi turned nine. All through her hospital stay that past spring, we'd paged through a book about New York City for kids, planning a visit there in the summer. She'd always wanted to see the Statue of Liberty in person, and the planning had been an especially good diversion during blood draws, changes of IV needles, and other unpleasant hospital business. In the end, the best time to travel turned out to be the day of Sammi's ninth birthday.

Wearing a soft blue dress and a pink zippered hoodie, she sat on the vents by the window of the airport clutching a Starbucks peppermint hot chocolate—I surmised that she'd learned to love this drink through osmosis in the womb—and grinning. I'd made her a giant pin with the words "It's My Birthday!" on it, and everywhere we went, people wished her happy birthday: on the flight, in the taxi to our rented apartment, and all through Central Park, where she was delighted by a balloon vendor who handed her a gigantic rainbow creation—"on the house!"—which she carried as she scampered up and down the hills.

We spent the week in New York in sensory delight—seeing, hearing, smelling, and definitely eating everything we could take in. The tiny counter of the apartment we were renting right above Times Square began filling with our leftover nibbles and bites—bagels and candy and greasy bags with the remnants of pastries—but of all the things we tried, the food we brought back from our ad hoc culinary tour of the Lower East Side was the biggest edible success of the trip.

I'd been especially excited to tour the Lower East Side because my mother had always spoken rhapsodically about the food she grew up eating in her Jewish Brooklyn home in the 1940s and 1950s. Her parents' house served as the center of family life for both sides when she was a child, and every Sunday had included a traditional Jewish deli brunch hosted by her parents and attended by aunts and uncles and cousins. She described trays full of bagels, platters of lox and cream cheese and tomatoes and onions, piles of rugelach and kichel, and blocks of halvah, with family crowding around the table, jostling and joking and putting their noses in everyone else's business. She wavered over the years about whether she enjoyed the raucous nudging and nosiness and tumult of those weekly brunches, but she never described the food with anything other than fondness. Chicago had some decent Jewish delis but nothing really compared to what was available in New York.

With most of my mother's family no longer in Brooklyn, I figured the best place to visit for classic Jewish American food would be the Lower East Side. We knew that we had to get bagels at Russ & Daughters, the famous deli, and I was lucky enough to find dairy-free cream cheese there, too. We collected an assortment of bagels and cream cheese, plus two cans of a sentimental old favorite: Dr. Brown's cream soda. Just a sip took me back to my high school years working in one of Milwaukee's only Jewish-style delis, where I often plopped down on an overturned bucket near the oven to eat a still-warm bagel and drink a can of this very treat.

Before we looked for somewhere to sit and eat, we walked just a few doors away, stepping into the heart of culinary nostalgia: Yonah Schimmel's Knish Bakery, a storefront and interior established in 1910 and seemingly barely changed in the hundred-plus years since. Knishes were a food of legend for me. According to my parents, there were no good places in the Midwest to buy a knish.

"A real knish," my father had told me, "is so greasy that it soaks through the paper towel you're holding it in."

A knish is the Jewish cousin to the empanada, samosa, pierogi, and bao, a potato-and-flour dough stuffed with greasy fried mashed potatoes, onion, salt, and seasonings. I'd only ever seen frozen ones, but my online research indicated that these from Yonah Schimmel's were the real deal. I'd been trying not to pay much attention to Sammi's eating habits on this trip, but a part of me thought knishes would be a win for her: soft and salty, easy to chew and swallow. At her last checkup with Dr. Lynn, she'd told me that Sammi still needed to put on a few pounds, and Sammi's favorite fruits weren't really the best path. Inside Yonah Schimmel's "knishery," I scanned the interior, searching fruitlessly for a cookbook that would allow me to re-create them at home. We stepped up to the counter and chose two varieties—a sweet potato one that made me secretly roll my eyes, offended by anything not traditional— and a plain potato one.

Across the street, we found two park benches that backed up to some fenced-in basketball courts. It wasn't the most auspicious environment for introducing my daughters to the foods of their ancestors, but ambiance wasn't important. We settled ourselves in and unwrapped the white butcher paper around the bagels and knishes. David took a picture of me biting blissfully into my first bagel with schmear in decades, thanks to the nondairy cream cheese. My face lifted to the sun, I closed my eyes and felt the yielding crust of the bagel give way to chewy dough and then smooth, salty, sharp chive creaminess. I chewed and swallowed, fully awake to the sensations I'd been missing all those years. In silence, I ate half the sandwich, wanting to leave room for the knish, which was steaming on the seat next to me.

Nearby Sammi nibbled her half of the plain bagel with plain cream cheese she was sharing with David, but struggled to get her mouth around the whole thing. David took the top layer off, and she tried to eat the bottom part, but it didn't look like she was loving it. I called her to come sit near me.

"I think it's time for you to eat a real old-fashioned Jewish food you've never tried before," I said, patting her on the knee. "Want to share this knish with me?"

"OK," she said. "I'll have a bite."

I tasted it first, just to make sure it wasn't too hot; if the first bite wasn't just right, I knew she wouldn't eat any more. My teeth pierced the dough, which was firm and salty, my lips feeling the oil that soaked through. In the hot August sun, the warm potato filling should have been wrong, but it was wonderful: velvety and rich, the taste my mother described in her stories of summers on Coney Island where she bought them on the beach, a mouthfeel that promised a full belly of starch and fat to keep me satisfied for hours. Nearby, I could hear Ronni reject the sweet potato knish and return to her slice of pizza. Reluctantly, I pulled my face away and held up the traditional potato knish for Sammi. Ducking my head to her level, I held it between us.

"Let's take a bite together," I said.

And then we did, each of us biting off a corner, our foreheads inches apart. I held all my feelings in my mouth as we breathed together: the wonderful taste, the connection to my mother, the hope I had that this food might be the key. When I pulled away, I looked at her chewing thoughtfully and asked what she thought.

"It's good," she said, with the same downward look at her lap that told me that although she didn't dislike it, she didn't love it. This would not be the key to her culinary heart. Along with another bite of knish, I swallowed my hope.

"Can we open the pickles now?" she asked, turning to face David as she hopped off the bench.

"Sure," he grinned as he pulled the heavy bag from underneath his seat. We'd stopped first—before the bagels and the knishes—at The Pickle Guys, a store my friend Hilary had recommended. The floor of this store was full of giant orange barrels promising all kinds of pickled products, everything from radishes and carrots to onions and watermelon, plus—of course—several kinds of pickled cucumbers. Sammi had always loved pickles. The cold, wet texture was easy on her esophagus, I'd come to realize. At home, I'd always stocked the spicy Israeli pickles she loved alongside other brined foods that had become her favorites over the years. She loved all kinds of olives, sticking canned black ones on her fingers and chewing the meat off the pits of Kalamata olives. During the hardest months of her six-food elimination diet, we'd even purchased cases of whole hearts of palm, the wide yellowish tubes she'd peel apart and eat like string cheese. None of these foods was very calorie dense, but she loved them.

Once inside The Pickle Guys store, Sammi had danced in glee around all the barrels. "Do they have *spicy* pickles?" she'd asked.

"You want *spicy*?" one of the salesmen yelled. "Kid, we *got* spicy!"

He'd walked us through the store, looking at all the offerings while we tried to decide how much we could buy and carry around throughout the rest of our day in the city. In the end, laden with several half-pound containers of pickled carrots, tomatoes, baby corn, and cucumbers, we also carried out a plastic bag with four whole traditional pickles in it. Measured in strength by "new," "half-sour," "¾ sour" and "sour," we gambled on the strongest one.

Standing with our elbows set widely and bending at the waist, we each took bites of our pickles on the sidewalk in front of the store. In a series of photos, Sammi takes a bite, scrunches her face, takes another, leans farther forward still as the juice dribbles down her hand, and puckers all the muscles of her face. Somehow, she simultaneously grins— joyful even as every tendon in her neck strains with the effect of all that vinegary flavor.

"It's good!" she finally said, leaning forward again to suck even more juice from the dripping pickle.

And so, after several bites of a bagel with schmear and two half-hearted nibbles of a knish, Sammi stood in front of a buffet of pickles, dipping fingers into plastic containers of pickled tomatoes and sliced cucumbers, enthusiastically slurping them as though only vinegar and garlic could sustain her. I watched, the grease of the knish on my lips, and kept quiet. *At least she's eating something.*

The next night, after another day of adventure in the city, we all went to see the musical *Matilda*. I'd read the book with Ronni years before, but Sammi didn't know the story of the smart, plucky, slightly telekinetic little girl who rose above her lot in life and chose her own destiny. I was prepared for both of my daughters to identify with the title character. What I did not expect, however, was how much determined little Matilda would remind me of myself.

In the second song of the show, "Naughty," Matilda sings about the characters in nursery rhymes and classic literature, frustrated by their fatalistic attitudes. She wonders why they don't just work to change the outcome of their stories instead of resigning to their fate. Though she was talking about Jack and Jill, Cinderella, and Romeo and Juliet, I heard myself reflected in her frustration. For years, I'd accepted Sammi's— and my—fate without much question.

In all the years of doggedly pursuing a better life for Sammi, I'd usually felt like an afterthought the minute I'd walked into a physician's office. They called me "Mom," as though there was nothing more to me than goodnight lullabies and carpool, never bothering to learn my name. They looked over my head, if they even looked my way at all, much more likely to be tapping at a keyboard with their back to me. They pooh-poohed my questions, handed me faded photocopies of recipes for the latest foods I'd have to make out of air and hope, and called me back to dispense test results that determined the fate of our lives without ever acknowledging the weight of their news or how long we'd waited to receive it. And still, through all of it, I'd been listening to my own instincts, pushing and trying and searching, and when I had heard enough, I refused a doctor's ridiculous idea for a therapy I knew wouldn't help, setting us on the path that led to Sammi's final surgery.

Sitting in the audience of *Matilda*, I listened to "Naughty" and watched little Matilda stick her hands on her hips and jut out her chin. She looked every bit as determined as I'd felt.

I reached over and took Sammi's hand. "Listen to that smart girl," I whispered.

She squeezed my hand in hers and whispered back, "I will."

After we returned home from our trip, I took Sammi for her last visit with her feeding therapist. To my surprise, in the two months she'd been in feeding therapy, she'd gained as much weight as she normally did in an entire year.

Something was working.

12

THE FIRST SANDWICH
IN A NEW WORLD

In the fall, Sammi started fourth grade, wherein all the most meaningful challenges were well within the realm of "normal" school escapades. She began learning to play drums in the school band; the Spanish immersion program in which she'd been enrolled since kindergarten started everyone in her class reading chapter books in Spanish; there was a mad rush to buy new soccer cleats when her pair from the previous season didn't fit the day before her first practice. She had homework and Sunday school, ukulele lessons and favorite TV shows. For the first time, Ronni didn't want to share her friends with Sammi as much as she had before, and we navigated closed doors and "big girls only" movie nights. It was all audaciously normal, and I marveled at all the time we had to manage it now that we were at the end of all the doctors' appointments.

Added to the time saved by making regular old food and Sammi's ever-improving speed in finishing her meals was the end of the process of carefully weaning her off her medication. This time, instead of abruptly stopping her PPI, we'd taken four months to cut her dose down slowly. She'd gone from her full dose, to three quarters of a dose, to half, to a quarter, to an eighth, and, finally, about a week before her annual physical, to skipping it entirely. When we went to see Dr. Lynn in October, Sammi had been off her medication for five days. After she'd been weighed and measured and checked, Dr. Lynn asked her a series of questions:

"Do you eat your vegetables?"

Sammi nodded. "Especially peas!" she said. "And also broccoli and brussels sprouts and tomatoes."

"Good!" Dr. Lynn turned to wink at me. "And not too much sugary soda and juice?"

"I don't like soda," she said, forgetting all the Sprite she'd drank in the hospital.

"OK then," Dr. Lynn continued. "And you sit in a booster seat in the car? And you always wear your helmet when you ride your bike?"

On and on it went, the same questions I'd recognized from Ronni's checkups, with Sammi nodding and answering seriously. When it was done, Dr. Lynn snapped the paperwork to the top of her clipboard and stood up.

"Well, Mom, she's a well child!" she grinned at me. "How's that sound for a change?"

"Pretty amazing," I admitted.

"I think this is really it, Sammi," Dr. Lynn said, holding up her hand for a high-five, which Sammi returned with a big smile. "No more surgeries and all that yucky stuff. Just go out and keep growing, OK? See you when you're ten!"

She left the room with a promise to send a nurse in with a flu vaccine. As soon as the door closed, I stood facing the exam table where Sammi was sitting and looked her right in the eye.

"Hey kiddo," I told her. "You are *well*. Your throat is healthy. Your ears are healthy. Your stomach is healthy. Your esophagus is healthy. Your heart is healthy. You are totally healthy!"

I wrapped my arms around her, the paper gown crinkling between us, and kissed the top of her head. When I pulled back, I saw that her eyes were brimming with tears. I held both of her hands and asked what was wrong.

She sniffled and said, "I've been different from everyone all the time, and now I'm not different anymore. It's weird."

A part of me crumpled inside, sick with the realization that we'd not impressed on her the other things that made her special. In all the years of strange diets and medicines and surgeries and doctors, how had we missed this?

"That's not really true, though," I told her. "You're still you, and you're more than just all this health stuff. Come on, tell me what some of the things are that make you Sammi, that make you special."

"Well," she said, "I'm creative."

"That's true!" I agreed. "You come up with so many good ideas!"

"And I'm silly. I'm the silliest person in our house."

"That's *definitely* true," I squeezed her hands. "You're really funny!"

"I'm nice to my friends."

"You sure are. You always want to make sure your friends are OK. What else?"

"I'm brave," she said with a sigh, as though she'd been holding onto that knowledge, relieved to finally admit it.

I agreed with her. "All that stuff is true; it really is. And now, you and I get to spend our time talking about that stuff and doing things to learn more about what you like and what you're good at and what you're curious about instead of spending all this time trying to help your body get healthy. Your body doesn't need all of our attention anymore, OK? That's what it means to be healthy."

She hugged me for a long moment, her head resting against my chest. I felt her breathing slow along with mine. After her flu shot, she picked out a sticker, and with that, we were done with her first ever well-child checkup.

Well child. I couldn't stop thinking about it the whole drive home and for days afterward. That's the term used to describe annual physicals that end like ours did—standard health advice for already-healthy children, a "well-child visit." But those visits had never ended that way for Sammi before. There had always been notes on the little slip of paper Dr. Lynn gave us to memorialize her measurements, instructions for two cups of Carnation Instant Breakfast per day, or to come back in six months for a weigh-in, or to follow up with a specialist, or to stay on her medication, or some other piece of advice that marked Sammi as not quite well. I didn't know how to trust the concept of Sammi as a "well child," but for some reason, this time it seemed easier than it had before. I had promised Sammi we would fill our lives with the stuff of well children. To do that with my whole heart, I had to give up my skepticism.

We plunged into autumn, a whirlwind of school and soccer and local children's theater. Because Ronni was in seventh grade and Sammi was in fourth, their Hebrew school sessions were at different times on the same day. Sammi was done at 6:15, just when Ronni started, and I decided that on the nights when David was traveling or working late, it didn't make sense to go home and make dinner, only to turn around and pick Ronni up again at eight. Instead, Sammi and I began a tradition of having a "Mommy-Sammi date" at our local Thai restaurant.

We'd settle into a table and pull out the giant menu even though we both always ordered the same thing: for me, the wide, fat noodles with tofu and broccoli called *pad sie eiu*; and for Sammi, *pad woon sen*: the thin, transparent "glass" noodles with scrambled egg, mushrooms, baby corn, and scallions. Her dish had very little seasoning, and the noodles offered barely any resistance to her teeth. We'd been ordering this dish for her for years as she'd struggled with the heavier gravies and sauces of other Thai noodle dishes. For our first two Thai food dates, she'd balanced her homework on the table while we waited for our food and then ate her *pad woon sen* distractedly, taking most of it home to eat from a thermos in her lunch box for the next several days. We had a great time together on these "dates," giggling about things that had happened at school or during my day of people watching while I worked at the coffee shop.

On the third visit, though, Sammi asked if she could try some of my tofu. I was elated—she seldom asked to try anyone else's food—but I tried to act casually as I spooned two pieces of it onto her plate.

"Mmmm," she said, chewing the first one thoughtfully. "This is really good!"

"I'm glad you like it," I said, the understatement of the last decade. Tofu, a protein-dense and infinitely adaptable food, was something I'd wished she'd eaten for the last several years. "Want some more?"

"Sure," she said, and I restrained myself from pushing my whole plate across the table at her. Instead, I picked out half a dozen pieces and set them on her plate. Along with half of her dish of *pad woon sen*, she ate all the tofu out of my dish.

"I don't want to take away all your food," she protested as I gave her more and more pieces.

"No, it's OK," I lied. "I like the noodles best anyway."

The next time we went, I asked Sammi if she wanted to try the dish I'd shared with her the last time.

"Actually," she said, shyly, "Can I get what Ronni always has?"

Ronni didn't like Thai food, actually. She'd subsisted on cold spring rolls on most of our outings to Thai restaurants for years, which was one of the reasons I'd chosen Thai food for my dates with Sammi, when Ronni wouldn't be sad to miss it. During the last year, though, Ronni had asked this particular restaurant if they would make their sweet-and-sour chicken (not really a Thai dish at all) as sweet-and-sour tofu. The result had added one more item on the menu that she tolerated. Now Sammi wanted to try it.

When it arrived in front of her, it was still steaming. I showed her how to put a little pile of rice on her plate and mix the sauce and breaded tofu into it, adding the chunks of onion and red bell pepper on the side. When she took her first bite, she pretended to faint out of her chair then came to, rhapsodizing about how delicious it was. For the first time, unprompted, she started talking with me about why it was good, discussing her food like a nine-year-old restaurant critic.

"It says sweet and sour because it really is, like, sweet *and* sour, at the same time!" she proclaimed. "And then the tofu is kind of hard on the outside but it's squishy on the inside, and the sauce squirts into my mouth when I bite on it. And when I need a break from the tofu I can eat the peppers cuz they're crunchy and even sweeter with the sauce."

I kept nodding, marveling at what she noticed. I wondered if she'd always noticed these things about her food, thinking not just about how it tasted but *why* it tasted that way. When I thought about it, I remembered little things she'd said before: how soft blueberries were juicier and the flavor went all over her mouth; how when she said "spicy" pickles, she really meant *flavorful* pickles, because the collection of dried herbs in my cabinet were called "spices" and added *flavor* to our food; how she liked matzo balls because they were "juicy," the broth in which they cooked soaking and saturating each spongy bite. While I had been watching her eating from the perspective of nutrition, she had, in her way, always paid attention to the flavor. Somehow, I'd missed this.

With all the emotional space for these conversations suddenly uncluttered by my worry, I started listening more closely to everything she was saying. I'd always thought I was a respectful parent, curious to know what my children wanted and needed, but I saw quickly that—in some ways, just like Sammi's doctors—I'd been taking care of Sammi's body far more than I'd been taking care of Sammi as a maturing, introspective human being. Though all the things I'd told her in the pediatrician's office about what made her special were true, there was more to learn about her.

One morning, she seemed extra tired. When I asked her if she'd had trouble sleeping, she said she'd waited until really late for the cat in her window. Since we didn't have a cat—and her window was on the third floor—I pressed her.

"What cat, sweetie?" I asked.

"The cat next door," she said. "She sleeps in the parking lot at night, but she wasn't there when I went to bed. I watched out the window for a long time but she didn't come. I hope she's OK."

I hadn't known that Sammi looked out her window for the cat at night or even that she could see into the neighboring apartment building's parking lot. "Is it a new cat?" I asked.

"No, she always lived here. Except in winter. Maybe she has a house for winter," she mused. "I hope she comes back tonight. I like to look at her before I go to sleep."

My little daughter had a relationship—in her mind, at least—with a stray cat, enough that she mused about its winter home, enough that she stayed awake to watch and wait for it to arrive. Everything about that charmed me, and I was impressed that she had not come down in the night to ask for help finding the cat or to admit her struggle to sleep without her nightly communion with her feline friend. Who was this fascinating little girl of mine? How had she navigated her emotions all this time while I watched her food intake and her size? I was about to find out.

Sammi seemed to notice that I had I taken my attention away from her diet and attached it to the rest of her, and our conversations blossomed into a fairy tale of parenting. That year, Ronni left for middle school by herself each morning half an hour before Sammi needed to leave for elementary school. Though I missed the three of us walking together as we had for all the years since Ronni had started kindergarten, there was beauty in walking alone with Sammi. She and I talked about all sorts of things now. She told me about her classmate and how much she loved his smile; about her plans for movies she wanted to make with her friend Sophie; about her favorite songs to sing in our synagogue's children's choir. We considered what she might learn next on the ukulele, discussed what it was like for me to grow up with a brother instead of a sister like she had, and mused about dressing up her pet lizard in hats and capes. It was as though the universe sent a new daughter for me and a new mother for her, familiar but far more fascinating than the ones we'd had before.

During the lulls between projects for my freelance work and while the children were at school, I explored my kitchen again, remaking my pantry for what felt like the tenth time. As I sorted through the ingredients from our past, certain I'd reject most of them, I found myself strangely nostalgic. I held each one in my hand, evaluating it with a mixture of sadness and curiosity. Did these things still have a place in our life?

I started with the baking cabinet, bringing out all the ingredients I had stored there onto the counters, spread out like a culinary history: the chickpea flour we'd made into flatbread and the dairy-, soy-, and nut-free powdered milk that went into the wildly complicated challah recipe we'd made during the most restrictive phase of the six-food elimination diet; the rice flour we'd used to thicken the sauce in my magic "safe" macaroni-and-cheese casserole; the tapioca starch that the homemade gluten-free flour blend had required. There were half a dozen packets of Jello and allergen-free decorative sprinkles. There was a dark quart-sized bottle of MCT oil, an ingredient I'd never understood that, somehow, was safe on the fat-free diet the previous spring.

Alongside the specialty ingredients were the ones I would have recognized before these diets: baking soda and powder, cornstarch, chocolate chips, brown sugar. I had extracts in half a dozen flavors, food coloring, cocoa powder, bags of shredded coconut, and blocks of baking chocolate. Arrayed on the counter like a mismatched army ready to stand against a hungry enemy, my ingredients seemed to wink and beckon. They told the story of days at the stove and the oven trying to fashion a little girl out of sugar and air and chemicals, fire and motion. They made my mouth shut against the grit of a cookie that didn't taste right but might be edible enough. I held each one in my hand before deciding whether continuing to own it would bring more pain or utility.

In the end, I kept the chickpea flour and released the rice flour, kept the tapioca starch and tossed the allergen-free sprinkles. I flipped through cookbooks in my mind, my eyes closed as I clutched a packet of xanthan gum, searching for its use in a world that now contained the gluten it had been purchased to replace. In the end, I threw it out. With glee, I poured the $40 bottle of MCT oil down the drain, never wanting to cook with it again. After wiping them clean, I reorganized my cabinets.

We were starting over, my kitchen and me, and this time, somehow I knew that our relationship had found its center.

One morning near the end of October found me scrambling for the makings of school lunches as the girls sat at the counter and ate their cereal in front of the iPad we'd bought before the surgery. Their oblivion to my frenzied poking into cabinets and refrigerator shelves started to frustrate me.

"Hey, guys, can you turn that off?" I finally snapped.

Reluctantly, they did.

"We are low on everything; I have to go to the grocery store later today. We're out of yogurt and tortillas; Ronni, would you eat a sandwich?"

Neither of my kids really liked sandwiches, unfortunately. Ronni had gone through a rice cake phase and a summer roll phase, and lately she'd been eating yogurt. Sammi, true to form, had stuck with black bean quesadillas. None of those things were options that day.

"Fine," Ronni sighed. "Can I have Safta's kind of sandwich?"

She was referring to my mom, whose dislike of peanut butter had made her sandwich of choice unique. In a world of PB&Js, my mother stood alone in preferring cream cheese and strawberry jelly. To me, her sandwich tasted like a slightly less-sweet cheesecake, not unlike the decadent creamy cheesecakes she had made and sold for several years when I was a little girl. I'd remembered this sandwich a few years earlier when Ronni had admitted that she only really liked peanut butter if it was accompanied by chocolate.

"Sure, I can make you Safta's sandwich," I said to Ronni. I rummaged through the fridge and found a tub of cream cheese. As I began to spread it on whole wheat bread, I wracked my brain for a lunch idea for Sammi. We had run out of tortillas, but we still had refried beans and cheese . . . unless. . . .

"Hey, Sammi," I asked hopefully, my back to her, "would you want to try this sandwich, too?"

There was a pause in which I thought I could almost hear her tapping her pointer finger on her chin as she considered my question. When the answer wasn't an immediate "No thank you," my heart pumped several extra beats. When she said, "OK, I'll try it," every molecule in my body vibrated as though I'd downed several shots of espresso.

"Sounds good," I said, my back still turned so she couldn't see the huge grin on my face. I spread one slice of bread half with cream cheese and half with strawberry preserves and folded it over on itself. Ronni got a full sandwich and Sammi the half. Both got a little container of cheese crackers, another of grapes, and a little baggie with two Oreos in it. For what might have been the first time ever, two nearly identical lunches were packed and ready to go.

At the end of the school day, I found Sammi's lunch box by the back door and opened it. She had eaten at least two-thirds of the sandwich. It was the first time she'd eaten a sandwich in her entire life. When I asked her if she'd liked it, she said she had and asked if she could have it again tomorrow.

For the next two weeks, I gave her half a cream cheese and jelly sandwich every day in her lunch. She seldom finished it, but if I reminded her about it when she got home from school, she'd take it out of her lunch box and finish it as she did her homework.

"I can't believe I didn't like sandwiches before," she said one day as I made dinner, passing me her empty sandwich container from lunch. "They're so good!"

I gave her a little squeeze before she walked away. It seemed unnecessary to say what I was thinking, which was that she probably couldn't swallow a sandwich before now. I imagined a compacted bolus of bread and cream cheese trying to make its way past the twists and turns of her pre-surgery esophagus and mentally shut the image out of my head as quickly as it had surfaced. There was no point in thinking about that now. Now, she could eat it. Now, she did.

The next week, Sammi and I arrived at our synagogue for Hebrew school. The students from nearby elementary and middle schools often gathered in the sunny alcove on the first floor to eat a snack before class, and Sammi sat next to my friend Rebecca's daughter on a bench, chatting. I did the same with Rebecca a few feet away. My back was to the children, but a few minutes later, Rebecca grabbed my arm and whispered.

"Is Sammi eating a *sandwich*?" she asked.

I turned and looked. Of her own accord, Sammi had unzipped her lunch box, taken out the remainder of her sandwich, and was finishing it, her legs swinging under her, as she visited with her friends. Our friend

Christine stopped near us and followed our eyes in the direction of the children on the bench.

"Get out!" she said. "What is in that sandwich?"

Both of these women who knew Sammi's struggle well were as awed as I was. They were surprised by the sandwich, which I'd known about, but I was overcome by Sammi's realization that she was hungry and her instinct to take out the food she had on hand and eat it, all of her own volition. The three of us watched as she popped the last bite into her mouth, stuffed the container into her lunch box, and then jumped up when she heard the religious school director calling from the floor above that class was starting.

"Here, Momma," Sammi said, rushing over to me. "Can you take my lunch box?"

I leaned down to give her a kiss, smelling the strawberries and cream cheese on her breath. Along with her friends, she ran up the stairs to class.

"How about that!" Rebecca said.

How about it, indeed. Moments like this had been accumulating quietly for months. A week later, Sammi ate nearly an entire adult-size helping of sweet-and-sour tofu at the Thai restaurant. Sometime in early December, she declared her loyalty to a specific brand of boxed macaroni and cheese. These moments were revelatory, of course, but the real gifts of that fall and winter after her surgery were the moments of connection between us. Not unlike our walk-to-school conversations, these flashes of future joy and deepening affinity for each other were teaching me how to be her mother all over again.

One night over dinner, we decided it would be fun to translate into Spanish the rascally rhyme about flatulence that I'd taught her from my own childhood. "Beans, beans," became "*frijoles, si*," and "the more you fart" became "*te tiras pedo tal*." We sat across from each other at our Thai restaurant, looking up translations on my phone and laughing so hard we could barely eat. I trusted she wouldn't share it in school, where half her classmates were native Spanish speakers, and we hoped the waitstaff didn't understand us either. As we practiced reciting our translation—which we knew might not be quite grammatically correct—we laughed even harder.

"You're the best mommy ever," she said as we walked out the door, our sides aching.

"That's definitely my goal," I answered her as I unlocked the car. "After all, I've got to match the best daughters ever."

It took me years to trust that Sammi was really and truly well, but the gradual belief in her health came with the richest rewards I could have asked for. We talked about poetry after her class read a book in verse; sitting on the couch, holding hands, I read her my favorite poem by E. E. Cummings, "i thank You God for most this amazing." Her eyes were wide as she told me it was beautiful. We admired flowers, squatted down to look closely at them, and we commiserated about how we both liked to sleep under a lot of blankets in a cold room so that we could feel the cool air on our faces. She, like me, worried about her friends if they were sad, coming down from her room at night to talk with me, cuddled close on the couch, about how to help them. When the boy in her class who'd begun picking on her the year before persisted, she told me that she didn't want to get him in trouble even if he deserved it. Like me, she was disinclined to disturb the social balance, forever bellyaching about doing the wrong thing.

Too, we learned that she loved stand-up comedy just like David and I did, and we searched for clean comedy for her. Watching her laugh at Ellen DeGeneres's 1996 album was even more fun than listening to it ourselves—she laughed with her whole body, throwing herself backward on the couch and banging the cushions with her fists. It made me recall a much tinier version of her, laughing at the Curious George movie while perched on a cushion on the floor, falling backward onto her back when her laughter overtook her. She'd been in there the whole time, I realized, this joyful creature hiding under her hunger and my nagging.

And as for me, my chef's skills honed under the most pressing circumstances, I realized that cooking had gone from a weight on my shoulders to—most days—a summoning finger, inviting me into an exciting unknown place. I experimented even further, exploring the Korean grocery store for new kinds of tofu and fresh ramen noodles, a dozen kinds of mushrooms, and carrots so big I could barely wrap my hand around their circumference. I tried new spices: yellow saffron I pulled apart with tweezers to bloom red into a ramekin of warm water;

the Middle Eastern spice blend called za'atar, with its oregano, thyme, sumac, and sesame seeds; and a bright plastic bottle of Tajín like the ones some of Sammi's Spanish-speaking classmates carried in their lunch boxes, full of a mixture of chilis, lime, and salt.

Even more profound were the moments I had started to accumulate when I prepared food just for myself. In all the years I'd been a parent, I'd seldom thought about taking time to make something just for me. I was a grabber-on-the-go, eating a scone and mocha at Brothers K Coffee House but never making breakfast for myself at home. If I wanted a snack before picking the girls up from school, it was usually something leftover, or a handful of tortilla chips, cashews, or two Oreos as I raced to the next stop in my day. But one early afternoon that first winter after Sammi's last surgery, I spied a mango on the counter. It was a favorite fruit for all four of us, and I usually chopped one up and handed a bowl full of mango chunks to the girls to eat after school. If it was something they liked, normally I never would have taken it for myself. I would have worried that it would be the one thing Sammi was willing to eat that day, and to be safe, I would have left it for her.

But that day, with a sensation that felt almost subversive, I cut it up just for myself. I put it in my favorite bowl—a hand-painted one I'd made for myself at a pottery shop with Sammi and a friend earlier that year—and took it to the kitchen counter. Delicately, I put the first bright, smooth bite into my mouth and felt the juice run over the sides of my tongue. I realized as I ate that I had had a mango to myself only a few times in my marriage, mostly on vacations to Mexico, where I'd buy a mango on a stick, covered in lime juice, salt, and chili powder. Chewing in my silent kitchen, I closed my eyes and remembered the first bite of mango I'd ever eaten, shared by David, who introduced me to the fruit in our first house in Chicago. I remembered the moment—married just two years, no children in sight—learning a new flavor from this man I loved, anticipating the sweetness of our life together, the mystery of the years to come. Now, bite after bite, alone in my quiet house, I filled my belly with a flavor that reminded me of being my own person, of being cared for.

How strange that I hadn't done this in years, I thought. Slowly, over the course of the months to come, I began making food for myself when my children were at school. I started with fruit cut up just for me—

apples with peanut butter, a bowl of sliced strawberries—and moved on to oatmeal I made on the stovetop with sliced peaches or blueberries, brown sugar, and nuts. The more I made things just for me, the more I felt safe and justified in making food for my family based on my own whims and tastes. Finally, I was freed not just from the dietary restrictions of Sammi's long medical journey but from my own instinct to serve others before myself.

Most sacred to my sense of love through food was my weekly baking of challah, connecting me to my friend Hilary, to my mother, and to a long tradition of Jewish women who made challah as a sacred act to welcome the Sabbath, setting the thumping of dough to the rhythm of the week. At the end of every school week, I mixed the dough for challah and set it to rise in the oven before picking Sammi and Ronni up from school. When we came in the door, the smell of yeast and sweet dough greeted us instantly.

"Mmmm, challah," they'd both say, eyes closed and noses sniffing.

One week Sammi stopped then, wrapped her arms around me, looked up into my face, and said, "Thank you for making challah every week."

"You're welcome!" I answered. "I love making it."

"And thank you for making such yummy food, too," she said, sighing, resting her cheek against my chest. "I love your food."

I thought, then, about the chickpea soup I spooned into her tiny mouth when she was a baby, about the mountains of blueberries and the piles of gluten- and egg-free pancakes, about the uneaten quesadillas and the gallons of Carnation Instant Breakfast, about the fat-free sushi and the Junior Mints, and I closed my eyes. Behind them lingered the food I'd begun to treasure: frittatas stuffed with broccoli and potato, Vietnamese summer rolls with tofu and sweet rice and basil leaves, chocolate-covered Oreos rolled in crushed peanuts, warm bread, pasta with butternut squash and vegan ricotta, enormous salads with vegetables of every color, foods we made for flavor and fuel, love and joy. I pressed my lips into Sammi's soft hair, thickening by the week, smelling of shampoo and spring breezes and something deeply linked to the chemistry of my own body.

I answered, finally and truthfully, "I love my food, too."

EPILOGUE

Nearly eight years after Sammi's final cardiac surgery, she's an entirely different person.

At sixteen, she is often mindlessly snacking at the kitchen counter, scrolling through social media as she pops still-frozen peas or malted milk balls or tortilla chips smothered in shredded cheese into her mouth.

"Hey, slow down," I tell her. "I'm about to start making dinner."

She weathered the pandemic either staring at her computer through endless Zoom meetings or walking, masked, with her friends to my beloved Brothers K Coffee House for her new favorite food: spinach-and-feta hand pies, which they toast for her to nibble on her way home. She discovered them after the local breakfast tacos shop closed, leaving her nearly in tears. Every week, when we have our "takeout Tuesday" meals, she begs for burritos or tacos. When we order from the one pizza place that will make me a pizza with nondairy cheese, she orders a giant grilled vegetable sandwich dripping with mayonnaise; when I am in the mood for Korean *ramyun*, she pants and sweats but eats the spicy vegetable noodle soup right alongside me. During the worst of the pandemic, we ate dinner every night in front of the TV, having spent the whole day together.

Sometimes I forget that I once had to beg her to eat.

Most of the time, though, I remember it, at least in pieces. When a friend told me that her child had been diagnosed with celiac disease, I recommended wholeheartedly the King Arthur Flour gluten-free mixes and the challah-shaped mold pan we used to make gluten-free challah, searching online for the links and emailing them right away. When a family member with a serious food allergy comes for dinner, I boil water to pour over every surface of my food processor before I use it to make anything she'll eat, scrubbing between the blades with a stiff brush, just in case. When a friend of mine was diagnosed with eosinophilic esophagitis, I offered to go to the grocery store with her, and when we did, I felt a secret exhilaration with every safe food we found; I just wanted to ease her way.

Now I am often the person my friends and family turn to when their health sends them down a path that includes dietary restrictions.

"What's something you're really going to miss?" I ask. "Let's see if we can re-create it."

It is thanks to the community around me—and Sammi—that we emerged on the other side of our medical journey with so much resilience and gratitude. I owe everything to my friends Andrea, Hilary, Christine, Clare, Amy, Ben, Rebecca, and Rina, plus dozens of others who did everything from wearing pink (symbolizing a smooth, pink esophagus) on the days of Sammi's endoscopies to showing up at our house with fruit and craft projects and DVDs when she came home from the hospital. The circle of women who shared their own vulnerabilities and the tapestry of their love always—but especially during the worst of the six months before Sammi's last surgery—kept me floating to the surface. My and David's families showered love on Sammi, which is what I needed from them most. David, the love of my life, kept pages of notes and did mountains of dishes and absorbed millions of my tears. We were scared, but we were never alone.

As I make the foods we love now, I remember sipping soy milk hot chocolate in my car when Sammi was a baby; sharing blueberries with Ronni and Sammi at the farmers market; making my grandmother's kugel; and sitting at Christine's dining room table in front of a plate full of safe-for-Sammi lentils and rice. I felt held, loved, and nourished in body and spirit. During all the hurt, the worry, and the struggle of those years, there were moments of grace that I now remember as a hand held out in the darkness. It's my turn to extend that hand.

I can't promise that every story of a child's labored eating will end as ours did. Sammi's experience was extraordinary. For every lucky child like Sammi, there are dozens who end up with further limitations due to allergies or eosinophilic disorders or other conditions. I can't even promise that the families of those children will find joy in eating the way we did even amid these diets; sometimes, food is little more than fuel. But I can promise that it's worth considering which battles to fight, which doctors to trust, and what deeper life lies beneath the medical issues your child is facing.

My family's peaceful life together is more valuable than any muffin recipe.

For more information on eosinophilic esophagitis:
American Partnership for Eosinophilic Disorders: https://apfed.org
National Organization for Rare Disorders—Eosinophilic Esophagitis: https://rarediseases.org/rare-diseases/eosinophilic-esophagitis/

For more information on double aortic arch and vascular rings:
Conquering CHD: www.conqueringchd.org
Mended Little Hearts: https://mendedhearts.org

For more information on feeding therapy:
American Speech-Language-Hearing Association: www.asha.org/public/speech/swallowing/feeding-and-swallowing-disorders-in-children/
Feeding Matters: www.feedingmatters.org

INDEX

ABOUT THE AUTHOR

Debi Lewis holds a BA and an MA in English and creative writing from the University of Wisconsin, where she was a recipient of the Eudora Welty prize for fiction. Her short fiction and essays have appeared in more than a dozen publications including the *New York Times, Huffington Post, Bon Appétit, Eureka Literary Magazine, Hippocampus, Kveller, Scary-Mommy, The Manifest Station, Brain Child Magazine,* and more. She has told stories in live storytelling events including Chicago's *This Much Is True, StoryLab,* and *The Moth.*

In 2005, Debi's second daughter's birth began what would become nearly a decade-long journey through the confusion and inefficiencies of modern pediatric specialty medicine, each step of which involved challenges with feeding. As she learned to cook for a variety of specialized diets, she came to love preparing food in a way that surprised and delighted her.

Debi Lewis lives in Evanston, Illinois, with her husband and two teenaged daughters. She runs a website design business and enjoys cooking, reading, and playing old-time fiddle. You can learn more about her at www.debilewis.com and follow her on Twitter at @growthesunshine.